Advancing Practice in Rehabilitation Nursing

Edited by

Rebecca Jester

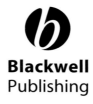

Blackwell
Publishing

© 2007 by Blackwell Publishing

Editorial offices:
Blackwell Publishing Ltd, 9600 Garsington Road, Oxford OX4 2DQ, UK
Tel: +44 (0)1865 776868
Blackwell Publishing Inc., 350 Main Street, Malden, MA 02148-5020, USA
Tel: +1 781 388 8250
Blackwell Publishing Asia Pty Ltd, 550 Swanston Street, Carlton, Victoria 3053, Australia
Tel: +61 (0)3 8359 1011

First published 2007 by Blackwell Publishing Ltd

ISBN: 978-1-4051-2508-6

Library of Congress Cataloging-in-Publication Data
Advancing practice in rehabilitation nursing / edited by Rebecca F. Jester.
p. ; cm.
Includes bibliographical references and index.
ISBN: 978-1-4051-2508-6 (pbk. : alk. paper)
1. Rehabilitation nursing–Quality control. I. Jester, Rebecca F.
[DNLM: 1. Rehabilitation Nursing. WY 150.5 A244 2006]
RT120.R4A38 2006
610.73′6–dc22
2006014909

A catalogue record for this title is available from the British Library

Set in 10/12.5 pt Palatino
by Graphicraft Limited, Hong Kong
Printed and bound in Singapore
by Markono Print Media Pte Ltd

The publisher's policy is to use permanent paper from mills that operate
a sustainable forestry policy, and which has been manufactured from pulp
processed using acid-free and elementary chlorine-free practices. Furthermore,
the publisher ensures that the text paper and cover board used have met acceptable
environmental accreditation standards.

For further information on Blackwell Publishing, visit our website:
www.blackwellpublishing.com

Advancing Practice in Rehabilitation Nursing

To my father (Frank), my husband (Saeid) and my son (Ali) – thank you so much for your love and support.

Contents

Preface

In recent years there has been an increase in the number of people in the UK requiring rehabilitation. This situation is not unique to the United Kingdom and colleagues internationally will find the issues discussed in this text relevant to their practice. The genesis of rehabilitation services has been, in part, a response to the recognition that maximising the quality of life and independence of individuals following trauma, disease or enduring chronic illness benefits society as a whole, as well as the individual.

While the role of the therapy professions is well recognised and established in the field of rehabilitation, the role of the registered nurse in rehabilitation is less well defined. New ways of working to support patients with chronic long-term conditions (LTCs) and their families are needed and the National Service Framework for LTCs affirms this. Rehabilitation as a nursing specialism has emerged in recent years, with registered nurses studying toward specialist practitioner status in rehabilitation at graduate or post-graduate levels.

Advancing Practice in Rehabilitation Nursing is written by nurses working within clinical rehabilitation settings or as educators in the field and has an accessible style and format. The book is aimed primarily at nurses practising at or studying toward specialist and advanced levels within rehabilitation and chronic disease management, but other health care professionals within these fields will also find the book useful to underpin advancement of their practice. The scope of the book reflects the diversity of rehabilitation nursing, with the first six and the concluding chapter providing general principles of specialist rehabilitation practice which are applicable to all client groups.

The remaining chapters are condition-specific and comprise examples from each of the main categories of people requiring rehabilitation. Throughout the book the emphasis is on holistic management of rehabilitation patients and a specific chapter on support for informal carers is included. The text focuses on the rehabilitation of adults, from adolescence to older age. Each chapter includes a comprehensive reference list.

Contributors

Denise Barr BSc (Hons), MSc, RGN, Clinical Nurse Specialist in Palliative Care, Gloucestershire Royal Hospitals Foundation Trust

Nicki Bellinger MSc, DipHE, RGN, Consultant Nurse Critical Care, Robert Jones and Agnes Hunt Orthopaedic and District Hospital NHS Trust, Oswestry, Shropshire

Steve Booth BA (Hons), MA (Ed), RGN, ENB 219, Principal Lecturer, Faculty of Health and Social Care, University of the West of England, Bristol

Tara Chambers MSc, DipHE, RN, Formerly Clinical Nurse Manager, Stroke Unit, Gloucestershire Hospitals NHS Foundation Trust, presently nursing in Australia

Rosie Grove BSc (Hons), PGDip, Diploma in Neurology and Neurosurgery, RGN, Nurse Consultant for Complex Physical Disability, Evesham Community Hospital, Worcestershire

Rebecca Jester BSc (Hons), PhD, RGN, ONC, DPSN, RNT, Head of School, School of Nursing and Midwifery, Keele University

Debbie Peniket MSc, RGN, RM, RHV, Assistant Director of Nursing and Therapies, South Birmingham PCT, Moseley Hall Hospital, Birmingham

Chapter 1
The Rehabilitation Process

Steve Booth and Rebecca Jester

It would seem prudent to begin our journey to advance nursing practice in rehabilitation by establishing what is meant by the term 'rehabilitation', what type of patients require rehabilitation and, indeed, to consider how we arrived at where we are now. In an attempt to address these issues this introductory chapter includes discussion of the following:

- Defining rehabilitation in the context of contemporary society and health care.
- The rehabilitation process: assessment, goal setting, treatment planning and evaluation.
- What types of patients require rehabilitation?
- Disability and enabling environments.
- Multidisciplinary versus interdisciplinary team-working within rehabilitation.
- Origins of modern rehabilitation.

Defining rehabilitation

If there was one phrase in health care I could eradicate it would be: 'the patient's waiting to go to rehab'. How many times have we heard this during handover or at the end of the patient's bed on an acute unit? First, rehabilitation is a process and not a physical location, and, second, why and what are they waiting for? Most comprehensive definitions of rehabilitation conclude it is a goal directed process comprising a number of stages, which aims to restore individuals to their maximum potential following disease or trauma. Therefore this process should begin as soon as the patient is medically stable. The Royal College of Nursing (RCN) rehabilitation forum provides a comprehensive definition of rehabilitation suggesting:

> 'Rehabilitation is a client centered, active and creative process which involves adaptation to changes in life circumstances. It is a shared activity between client, carer and professionals who recognise the individual

contribution of all concerned. It is designed to enable the client to achieve optimum and/or acceptable level of functioning. Its aim is to minimise handicap resulting from impairment and/or disability.' (RCN 1994)

This definition affirms the importance of patients being active partners, rather than passive recipients, in the rehabilitation process and this may create a challenge to conventional views of nursing, where the nurse is seen as 'doing for' the patient what they are unable to do for themselves. However, rehabilitation nursing is concerned with maximising independence and this requires a more 'hands-off' motivational approach, which patients, their families and nurses themselves may find difficult to accept. More detailed discussion of appropriate models of nursing in rehabilitation can be found within the historical context section of this chapter and within Chapter 2. The RCN definition emphasises the important role of informal carers as partners in the rehabilitation process, and a fundamental aspect of advancing nursing has to be the support and preparation of family carers, which is discussed in Chapter 6.

The rehabilitation process

The rehabilitation process comprises a number of stages:

- Comprehensive assessment
- Setting of short-, medium- and long-term goals
- Development of a collaborative plan to work toward achieving the goals
- Evaluation of progress toward the goals

The process should be seen as cyclical with regular re-assessment, review and adjustment.

Comprehensive assessment

A key component of the advancing nursing role is that of holistic health assessment. Holistic health assessment aims to capture data in a systematic and comprehensive format and includes all aspects of the patient's well being, including: physical and mental health, psychological status, social circumstances, beliefs and aspirations for their health and well being. It is important that repeated assessment is avoided, and for this reason the multidisciplinary team must develop a shared assessment document that can be used by all members of the team. Also, it must be agreed who will be responsible for what aspects of collecting data, to avoid either repeating or missing important information and to maximise the full potential of the team. The shared assessment document should form an integral part of the patient's pathway of care and treatment, and so there should be the ability to build upon information elicited during the acute phase of the patient's journey. Integrated care pathways are an ideal framework to foster both seamless integration of the acute and rehabilitative phases and interdisciplinary working. There are various methods of collecting data during holistic health assessment, including:

- Observation – sensing, seeing or smelling
- Interview – including history taking
- Listening
- Consultation with other members of the multidisciplinary team, family members, patient's notes and hand-held records, etc.
- Physical examination, e.g. inspection, palpation, percussion and auscultation
- Assessing physical function, range of movement, gait and mobility, etc.
- Judicious use of clinical investigations
- Self-report measures of health and disease

A significant number of rehabilitation patients have communication difficulties, either due to problems with speech or cognitive dysfunction. Specialist support from the speech and language therapists should be used as appropriate, while liaison with family members can be useful to supplement information elicited from the patient. The most important aspect of the assessment is systematic and comprehensive history taking, with Silverman & Hurst (1996) suggesting an accurate diagnosis can be made on the history alone in 80% of patients. Clinical investigations should be judiciously requested to avoid any unnecessary discomfort to patients and waste of valuable resources. Investigations should only be ordered if their results will enhance the accuracy of diagnosis or influence treatment decision options.

Goal setting

For many nurses from non-rehabilitation backgrounds goal setting is a relatively new skill, as most models of nursing identify patient problems or needs, rather than developing goals. In many established rehabilitation centres regular goal setting and review meetings are held with active participation of the patient and their family members. This is highly appropriate because the goals must be relevant and specific to each individual's unique situation. Goals should be realistic and achievable, but at the same time provide a moderate degree of challenge to the patient. Patients should be encouraged to set short-, medium- and long-term goals, as viewing relatively small targets as part of a longer term achievement can provide motivation. Realistic time scales need to be set for each goal and interim points for review of progress agreed with the patient.

Development of a collaborative plan to work toward achieving the goals

As an integral part of the goal setting process a plan of action needs to be developed and agreed between the patient, their family and the multidisciplinary team. Health care jargon should be avoided and the plan should be both comprehensive and understandable to the layperson. It must be agreed which member/s of the team has the best skills and expertise to support the patient with each particular goal. This does not negate the responsibility of other team members, but rather it helps to ensure coordination and clarity to the process. The treatment plan should be evidence-based wherever possible, and alternative approaches discussed with the patient and their family to ensure informed consent and cooperation. It is imperative that the patient's waking day is planned to maximise engagement in meaningful therapeutic activity that will contribute to the achievement of the goals.

The specialist nurse has a key role to ensure that all members of staff, including students and support staff, work toward the patient's agreed action plan. Even within established specialist units we still encounter a culture of 'getting the work done', which often results in staff doing things for patients, such as washing and dressing, as it is quicker than supporting them to do it themselves. Patient motivation plays a key role in the achievement of goals and there is nothing more frustrating than working with a patient who has the physical and cognitive ability to achieve, but lacks motivation. However, as will be discussed in Chapter 4, clinical depression can often go undetected in rehabilitation patients and clearly this will have a severe adverse impact on their motivation. Guthrie and Harvey (1994) suggest the following to maximise patient motivation:

- Information, to reduce threat and restore control
- Providing choice and participation in goal setting
- Attention to social and emotional needs
- Discouraging families from being over-protective
- Creating a therapeutic culture of optimism and hope
- Providing positive role models, e.g. patients with a similar injury or disease who have achieved success

Evaluation of progress toward the goals

Progress toward achievement of the patient's goals needs to be reviewed on a regular basis and should be a shared activity between the multidisciplinary team, the patient and their family. There are several aspects of progress evaluation, these include: the patient's own self-reporting; physical measurements, such as timed walking, range of joint movements; disease-specific and general quality of life indices, e.g. Barthel Index, Rivermead Mobility Index; and multidisciplinary team reports based on observation and interaction with the patient. Detailed discussion of evaluation methods in rehabilitation is provided in Chapter 5. The patient, their family and the multidisciplinary team should review the triangulation of these sources of evidence and discuss issues of partial attainment and any potential barriers hindering progress. Based on this discussion the patient's goals and action plan should be reviewed and amended as appropriate.

What types of patients require rehabilitation?

The demand for rehabilitation services will continue to increase due to a number of factors, including: dramatic changes in the demography of illness and disability due to the increasing incidence of chronic diseases; a rise in the proportion of older people; as well as serious disability and suffering caused by war and terrorism. Those conditions requiring rehabilitation can be categorised as follows:

- Acute onset, e.g. stroke and myocardial infarction
- Gradual onset/relapsing course, e.g. multiple sclerosis and rheumatoid arthritis
- Acute onset/constant course, e.g. spinal cord injury and traumatic amputation
- Gradual onset/progressive course, e.g. osteoarthritis and cardiac failure

It is highly probable that some patients will be suffering from several comorbid conditions and may meet the requirement for case management as well as rehabilitation services (please see Chapter 10 for further detail on case management). Rehabilitation services will continue to need to demonstrate cost-effectiveness and evidence-based practice, specifically in the context of the reconfiguration of commissioning skills-based services and a continual move toward community- and primary care-based provision (discussion on service evaluation can be found in Chapter 5). People requiring rehabilitation range from young children to older people, and an important aspect of advancing nursing practice in rehabilitation is to apply theoretical knowledge of the relevant physical, social and psychological stages of development to the individual child, adolescent, adult or older person. In the UK, rehabilitation services are often organised into child and adult provision, but this can lead to a period of uncertainty for adolescents who need support to make the transition from the child to adult services. We need to ensure that the pathways of referral from child to adult service are seamless and transparent and that there is effective communication between the teams.

Disability and enabling environments

Many of the people requiring rehabilitation services will have a disability, which may be permanent or temporary. In recent years there has been a recognition that disabled people are not a problem, the problem is the way society is organised to discriminate against those individuals with a disability. The Disability Discrimination Act 1995 has supported this social model of disability and prohibits less favourable treatment of people who have or who have had a disability. This Act gives new rights to disabled people in relation to:

- Access to goods, facilities and services
- Employment
- Buying or renting land or property

Disabled people should enjoy the same rights as able-bodied people, and the social model of disability considers what changes would be necessary so that people are facilitated to live ordinary independent lives. Disabled people have identified seven fundamental needs (Crosby & Jackson, 2000), which have to be met for independent living to be a realistic proposition:

- Information about choices
- Peer support and counselling
- Appropriate housing, which you can get into, move about in, live in and is in the right place
- Equipment to support you to do the things you want to do
- Personal assistance to facilitate independence
- Accessible transport
- Access to the built environment

As nurses aiming to advance rehabilitation practice we have a responsibility to ensure that: we provide the services to support the inclusivity of individuals with disability; we work with other members of the multidisciplinary team and social services to provide up-to-date information for our patients regarding their rights under The Disability Discrimination Act 1995; and we maximise enabling environments where rehabilitation is being carried out, be that within the tertiary or community setting.

Multidisciplinary versus interdisciplinary team-working with rehabilitation

One of the key skills needed in rehabilitation is team-working (Wade & de Jong, 2000), but we need to be clear that we understand what is meant by 'team-working' and also to be able to differentiate between multidisciplinary and interdisciplinary working. Pearson (1999) provides a useful comparison of multi- and interdisciplinary working, the principal differences are outlined in Table 1.1. There has been an increasing move toward interdisciplinary working in recent years and this is highly likely to continue with the implementation of skills-based commissioning of services. The important factors are that the team's collective skills and knowledge meet their clients' needs and that there is effective team leadership and communication. It is not appropriate in contemporary health care for a specific professional grouping to always be the team leader, but rather that the team leader has the appropriate skills and knowledge of leadership and coordination. Gibbon *et al.* (2002) identified a number of potential attitudinal barriers to effective interdisciplinary team-working, which

Table 1.1 The key differences between interdisciplinary and multidisciplinary team working.

Interdisciplinary working	Multidisciplinary working
• Patient oriented goals • Use of integrated pathways and documentation • Blurring of professional boundaries and more sharing of roles and responsibilities • Team leader not profession-specific, but based on skills and experience of team leadership and coordination	• Profession discrete goals • Each profession retains its own records for individual patients • Clearly demarcated role boundaries • Team leader tends to be a medic

included: professional jealousies and role boundaries; perceived loss of autonomy and threat to professional status; lack of knowledge and unrealistic expectations of the role of other professions. In addition, a number of practical obstacles may inhibit effective interdisciplinary working, which include: lack of time to attend team meetings; differing working patterns between the professions; and organisational separation of line management and professional accountability.

Take time to reflect on the team that you work with and analyse your current model of working in relation to interdisciplinary working and coordination, and, if appropriate, discuss and develop an action plan to maximise your team-working as this is an essential step in advancing practice in rehabilitation.

Origins of modern rehabilitation

To help us move forward with team-working and ultimately to advance our practice it is useful to explore the origins of modern rehabilitation.

To begin a history of rehabilitation with the statement 'there is no definite history of rehabilitation' seems to be a foolish act. The absence of a distinct chronology for rehabilitation, as there would be for say orthopaedics or neurosurgery, is a challenge. However, the values of recovery and recuperation have not been overlooked. Early writers and thinkers, such as Plato and Asclepius, understood the value of creating an environment for healing and also that the mind may aid the body to recover. Joseph Trueta speaking in 1963 notes that at Epidaurus in Greece there are indications of treatments inscribed on votive plaques and evidence of a gymnasium, baths, theatre and promenades that date from over 2000 years ago.

Trueta adds:

'Faith, beauty, peace, music, baths, exercises, sports, competitions and one or two light drugs: that was the only medicine known to our forefathers . . .

This is, almost exactly, the basis on which modern rehabilitation has been established.' (Trueta, 1963, p. 346)

Nursing theories and models in the context of rehabilitation

Henderson suggests that the holistic nature of nursing lays the foundation for nurses to be 'rehabilitators par excellence'. Holism and promoting patient independence have been central concepts to many nursing models. Roper, Logan and Tierney's model utilises a dependence/independence continuum that tries to explain that the person may be able to achieve health despite being disabled (Roper *et al.*, 1980). Maintenance of health involves assessment of the individual in the twelve activities of daily living (ADLs) and the influence on the ADLs of five factors, which are broadly recognisable as the external and internal factors of biology, psychology, sociocultural, environmental and politicoeconomic.

For some theorists it is the manipulation of these factors that allows the person to adapt to the stresses of the external and internal environments. Callista Roy's adaptation model (first published in 1970) stresses the balance perspective, with nurses seeking to manipulate or change the environmental stimuli to allow the person to adapt and thus achieve wellness (Roy, 1980).

Dorothea Orem took a unique perspective on the notion of the underlying focus of human endeavour and suggested that the drive for humans is to be self-caring. (Orem, 1980). The 'deficit' for Orem occurs when an individual is unable to self-care and requires an intervention that must be taken over by the nurse as the self-care agent. In several other models the nurse is the 'manager' of the holistic process for the patient – see, for example, Betty Neuman's (1982) model – that is to say, the nurse manages the individual and their complex systems to achieve a balance.

All nursing models, to some degree, have a sense of the wholeness of the individual where biological, sociological and psychological factors influence health. For nursing theorists there is a clear link between the individual and their environments, both internal and external, and there are clear links between the works of these authors and the rehabilitation goals of adjustment and adaptation to a condition or disease.

Rehabilitation and the professions

As nurses working within rehabilitation it is useful to understand the development of other professional groups within the specialty, as this may help us develop strategies to minimise professional rivalry and maximise interdisciplinary working in contemporary rehabilitation.

Physiotherapy developed as a discrete professional group when four nurses organised themselves to protect the name of massage nurses from the scurrilous reporting of the press. In the early years of the last century, massage nurses, later physiotherapists, began to develop a treatment typography distinct from that of the medical professions and that could lay claim to its own knowledge base. Using the recently developed electrical treatments and exercises, the proto-physiotherapist became an enabler of the physical recovery of the patient, coming into her own during First World War. In the USA the American Women's Physical Therapy Association (AWPTA) was formed in 1921; while, in the UK, the Society of Trained Masseuses, which had formed in 1895, received its Royal Charter in 1920.

The development of occupational therapy as a discrete professional group can be traced back to 1917, when the Division of Special Hospitals and Physical Reconstruction, formed by the US Surgeon General, became responsible for the training and management of reconstruction aides who were to assist disabled servicemen to return to active living. This Division was to become the forerunner of the occupational therapy profession. In the UK, Dr Elizabeth Casson established the first school of occupational therapy in Bristol during the late 1920s.

In the USA, R. Tait McKenzie, a physician who taught at the University of Pennsylvania Medical School, had worked to develop treatment regimes for disabled patients, which would be broadly recognised as physical therapy. McKenzie, a far-sighted individual also recognised the 'treatment by occupation'. Writing in his text *Reclaiming the Maimed*, published in 1918, he said:

'Treatment by occupation differs from all other forms already described in that the remedy is given in increasing doses with the patient's improvement. It is the final page in his progress, to which all others lead up.' (cited in Fishman, 2004)

From this brief historical overview we begin to see how physiotherapists and occupational therapists developed a level of professional autonomy within the field of rehabilitation; claiming a discrete knowledge and skill base from medicine.

War and industry as the catalysts for rehabilitation

It has often been said that conflicts across the world and centuries have led to changes in the organisation and provision of health care and the development of new treatments and techniques. An example is provided by Cooter (1993) who notes that the understanding of the causes of shell shock in the years after the First World War led to the screening of applicants for mental health problems during the Second World War, what Cooter calls 'the medicalisation of the mind'. This gave the impetus for the post-war developments in psychiatry.

Following the First World War there was a legitimate change in the approach to rehabilitation at a national level with the realisation, by the populations of all countries affected by the War, that disabled servicemen and -women could not be managed in institutions shut away from those that they had fought for.

These soldiers, sailors and airmen had sustained their injuries serving their country and deserved the country's support and aid. Plans had been made during the First World War to deal with the likely numbers of disabled servicemen. This level of state control and planning of the *ante-belum* world was quite new and required legislation to progress the cause. The inter-war years (1918–1939) are seen as the period of development of the rehabilitation specialty before further refinement and consolidation in the 1940s and later.

By the start of the Second World War, Cooter (1993) says that the 'success of rehabilitation was seen to depend upon the integration of services and different types of health care workers within geographical areas' (p. 199), and that rehabilitation was being talked of as the 'one fashion which dominates medical thought almost to the exclusion of any rivals' (Editorial, Medical Press and Circular 1943 – quoted in Cooter, 1993.).

In December 1941, Gladys M. Hardy, writing in the *British Journal of Nursing*, exhorting the young women of Britain to consider how best they could serve their country by nursing, suggested that they would:

'help in the glorious work of rehabilitation amongst those heroes to whom we owe our lives and homes.' (Hardy, 1941)

Clearly, war and conflict have heavily influenced the development of rehabilitation services in the western world. A further strong impetus to develop and organise rehabilitation services has been industry. Despite methods of caring for the injured and ill resulting from work and toil having existed for centuries, it took the creation of industrialised capitalism to refine the idea of the worker as an economic unit. Early industrial processes and machinery were dangerous and caused untold damage and death to workers. Engels, writing in 1845, notes:

'Besides the deformed persons, a great number of maimed ones may be seen going about in Manchester; this one has lost an arm or a part of one, that one a foot, the third half a leg; it is like living in the midst of an army just returned from a campaign.' (cited in Doyal p. 53)

Engels' analogy is entirely apposite, given the scale and the similarities of the workers' and soldiers' injuries and in returning them to work as quickly and efficiently as possible after injury.

Echoing the idea of the wastage of economic units, *The Lancet* in 1926 commented on the lack of continuing care for the worker who had been damaged as a result of his work. Writing of the purpose of the treatments in hospital, the author V. Warren Low (1926) pointed out the failings of the system and the need to create a different type of hospital:

'Whether the man makes any economic use of his restored function does not appear to be any concern of theirs. Industry would seem to require another kind of hospital, or what might be called an "after-care centre".' (cited in Cooter, 1993, p. 201)

Roger Cooter (1993) suggested that rehabilitation had emerged from the 1930s as a strong movement across all branches of medicine. Cooter's examination of the work of Ernest Nicholl (Director of the Berry Hill Rehabilitation Centre) and H.E. Moore (at Crewe) between the wars highlighted not only the impetus to return the worker to his work, but to reduce the vast sums in compensation by cutting the time between injury and return to the workforce (Cooter, 1993).

The influence of history on contemporary rehabilitation

From the 1950s rehabilitation continued to develop as a discrete specialty within medicine, but services tended to be geographically isolated from main health care provision within major cities, often being located in rural areas. This geographical isolation reflected the philosophical isolation, with rehabilitation being viewed as a completely separate entity to acute medicine rather than an inherent part of the patient's journey to recovery. In the early 1970s Royal Commissions attempted to raise the profile of rehabilitation by promoting the relocation of services to within district general hospitals (Smith, 1999). However, a significant shift in emphasis in how rehabilitation is perceived only really emerged after the introduction of the Community Care Act in 1989, which brought about a major reconfiguration in the way health services were commissioned and delivered. Furthermore, the economic realisation that the ageing population within the UK need to be supported to be as fit and independent as possible has prompted commissioners of health care to support further development of rehabilitation services, specifically in respect of specialist rehabilitation units within acute trusts, case management of people with chronic long-term conditions and community-based rehabilitation services being an integral part of mainstream community care.

The 1950s onward has seen the further development of physiotherapy and occupational therapy as professions with a specific and recognisable role within rehabilitation services, which has been supported by graduate level preparation for registration. Indeed, the contribution of therapists is so well established within rehabilitation in the twenty-first century that rehabilitation is often referred to as 'physio' or 'therapy'.

Nursing, to date, has not succeeded in firmly establishing its role within rehabilitation, and ambiguity about the nursing contribution continues to be debated. However, this text aims to explore and support the advancing role of nurses within rehabilitation and this is discussed in greater detail within the following chapters. History has taught us that nursing has always been there to support those requiring rehabilitation and the twenty-first century presents us with an opportunity to maximise our contribution, and to firmly establish our role and work in partnership with patients and other health care professionals to maximise the quality of rehabilitation services.

Conclusions

The similarity of the influence of both war and industry on rehabilitation stems from a necessity to maximise the usefulness of individuals to society and reduce the burden of injury and disability on the economy. However, rehabilitation as a vehicle to maximise the independence and quality of life of the individual must be viewed as of equal importance as the potential collective impact of rehabilitation on society as a whole. In addition, the realisation that the disabled individual is not the problem, but rather that the environment is not an enabling one has culminated in legislation to enable and prevent discrimination on the grounds of disability. This chapter has attempted to provide an introduction to advancing practice in rehabilitation and to provide an overview of the development of rehabilitation services. It is important for us to understand where the specialty has come from, specifically the development of discrete professional groups that comprise the multidisciplinary team.

References

Cooter R. (1993) *Surgery and Society in Peace and War. Orthopaedics and the Organisation of Modern Medicine 1880–1948*. London, MacMillan.

Crosby N. and Jackson R. (2000) *The Seven Needs and the Social Model of Disability*. Derbyshire Coalition for Inclusive Living.

Dale E.T. (1951) *Report of a Committee of Inquiry on Industrial Health Services*. Available from: www.bopcris.ac.uk/bopall/ref9471. [Accessed 28/10/05]

Department of Health (1989) *Caring for People: Community Care in the Next Decade and Beyond*. London, HMSO.

Engels F. (1845) *The Condition of the Working Class*. [Cited in Doyal L. (1979) *The Political Economy of Health*. London, Pluto.]

Fishman A. (2004) *Rehabilitation Medicine at the University of Pennsylvania 1914–1919*. Available from: www.uphs.upenn.edu/rehabmed/history/chap2 [Accessed 25/01/06]

Gibbon B., Watkins C., Barer D., Waters K., Davies S., Lightbody L. and Leathley M. (2002) Can staff attitudes to team working in stroke care be improved? *Journal of Advanced Nursing*, **40** (1), 105–111.

Guthrie S. and Harvey A. (1994) Motivation and its influence on outcomes in rehabilitation. *Reviews in Clinical Gerontology*, **4**, 235–243.

Gutman S. (1995) Influence of the US military and occupational therapy reconstruction aides in World War 1 on the development of occupational therapy. *American Journal of Occupational Therapy*, **49** (3), 256–262.

Hardy G. (1941) *British Journal of Nursing*, **201**, Dec.

Henderson V. (1980) Preserving the essence of nursing in a technological age. *Journal of Advanced Nursing*, **5**, 245–260.

Johnson D.E. (1980) The behavioral system model for nursing. In: *Conceptual Models for Nursing Practice*, 2nd edn (J.P. Riehl and C. Roy, eds). New York, Appleton-Century-Crofts, pp. 197–206.

Neuman B. (1982) *The Neuman Systems Model*. Norwalk, Conn, Appleton-Century-Crofts.

Orem D. (1980) *Nursing Concepts of Practice*, 2nd edn. New York, McGraw Hill.

Pearson A. (1999) The coordinating role of nursing within rehabilitation. In: *Rehabilitation in Adult Nursing Practice* (M. Smith, ed.). Edinburgh, Churchill Livingstone.

Roper N., Logan W. and Tierney A. (1980) *The Elements of Nursing: A Model Based on a Model of Living*, 1st edn. Edinburgh, Churchill Livingstone.

Roy Sr C. (1980) Adaptation: a conceptual framework for nursing. *Nursing Outlook*, **18** (3), 42–45.

Royal College of Nursing (1994) *Standards of Care: Rehabilitation Nursing. Rehabilitation Nurses Forum Committee*. London, RCN.

Silverman M. and Hurst W. (1996) *Clinical Skills for Adult Primary Care*. Philadelphia, Lippincott-Raven.

Smith M. (1999) *Rehabilitation in Adult Nursing Practice*. Edinburgh, Churchill Livingstone.

Stryker R. (1996) Foreword. In: *Rehabilitation Nursing. Process and Application*, 2nd edn. St Louis, Mosby.

Trueta J. (1963) Rehabilitation – past and future. *Physiotherapy*, **49** (Nov), 346–351.

Wade D. and de Jong B. (2000) Recent advances in rehabilitation. *British Medical Journal*, **320**, 1385–1388.

Warren Low V. (1926) Workman's compensation and the surgeon. *Lancet*, 23 Oct., 849–850. [Cited in Cooter R. (1993) *Surgery and Society in Peace and War. Orthopaedics and the Making of Modern Medicine, 1880–1948*. London, MacMillan.]

Chapter 2
The Role of the Specialist Nurse Within Rehabilitation

Rebecca Jester

The aim of this chapter is to explore the unique contribution of nurses and nursing in rehabilitation within the context of contemporary health care. The proliferation of specialist and advanced roles within rehabilitation nursing, both internationally and in the UK, will be discussed with specific reference to the development and implementation of such roles and the potential impact on service provision. Indicative content includes:

- The unique contribution of nurses within rehabilitation
- Advancing nursing practice – what does it mean?
- Spheres of professional practice: novice/primary/specialist/advanced
- Multi-faceted nature of specialist nursing – expert practitioner, consultant, educator, researcher, co-ordinator and change agent
- Nurse prescribing
- Professional autonomy and decision-making
- Implementing and evaluating advanced nurse practice roles

The unique contribution of nurses within rehabilitation

Chapter 1 highlighted the valuable contribution made by nurses and nursing to the specialty of rehabilitation, specifically during and following the First and Second World Wars. Rehabilitation nursing is not a new phenomenon, but there has been an ongoing discussion about what, if any, is the unique contribution nurses make to contemporary rehabilitation practice.

The contribution of therapists, social workers, physicians and psychologists is well defined within the rehabilitation process. However, the role of the nurse in rehabilitation is less clearly defined and nurses often find it difficult to articulate their unique contribution. Waters (1996) considered the role of nurses to be secondary and comprising three main components:

- General maintenance – including overall ward management and maintaining patients' physical well being in terms of nutrition, hygiene and skin care.

- Specialist – an inherent degree of expertise in areas such as tissue viability, continence and pain management.
- Carry-on-role – the nurse maintains the progress made by therapists, specifically in walking and dressing throughout the 24-hour period.

The roles outlined above clearly constitute a part of the nursing role within rehabilitation. They are important aspects of supporting patients to reach their rehabilitation goals. A patient who has unmanaged pain or is incontinent of urine when they stand is unlikely to be able to maximise their functional and mobility status. These factors will, of course, have a deleterious effect on their psychological well being leading to de-motivation, frustration and possible clinical depression. However, the secondary role outlined by Waters fails to take into account the complexity, depth and potential of nurses' roles within rehabilitation.

Twenty-four hour presence

Johnson (1995) suggested that nurses are in an ideal position to close the circle in the rehabilitation process, ensuring that new skills learnt in therapy sessions are incorporated into everyday life. Clearly, nurses are the only professional group within rehabilitation to provide a 24-hour service, 7 days per week, particularly within inpatient rehabilitation settings. The 24-hour presence provides nurses with a unique opportunity to not only reinforce new skills learnt and incorporate them into everyday activities, but to evaluate patients' progress at different times of the day and night. For example, it is not uncommon for non-nurse members of the multidisciplinary team to declare a patient fit for discharge based on snapshot assessments during the day, necessitating nurse members of the team to report important issues such as: the patient suffers with confusion, nocturia, uncontrolled pain and a tendency to fall, etc. during the night. A study by Ellul *et al.* (1993) reported that when nurses on a rehabilitation unit were educated to incorporate the skills patients learnt within therapy sessions into all aspects of patients' care, it resulted in an increase of 55% of the time patients spent engaged in meaningful therapeutic activity. This exemplifies the huge impact nurses can make within rehabilitation if they have the appropriate skills and knowledge.

Barriers to maximising the role of nurses in rehabilitation: changing attitudes

The change from the nurse doing things for the patient to encouraging self-reliance is one that nurses, patients and relatives all find difficult. The traditional definitions of nursing emphasise the role of the nurse in providing care for those too sick to care for themselves. As specialist nurses we have a key role to play in educating nurses, other members of the multidisciplinary team, managers, patients and their families to embrace a model of 'enlightened withdrawal' of support in rehabilitation nursing, with an emphasis on caring about, rather than caring for, patients. This requires a significant shift in both thinking and culture for nurses to feel comfortable with adopting a 'hands-off' approach to maximise patient independence, which requires a move away from a ritualistic 'getting things done' mentality.

One of the first practical steps we can take in shifting the attitudes and behaviours of nurses is to ensure that, as specialist nurses, we input into the development and delivery of both pre- and post-registration nursing curricula.

Potential role of nurses in rehabilitation

To date, in the UK, the role of nurses in rehabilitation generally remains underdeveloped. This may be partly due to a dearth of educational programmes designed specifically for post-registration nurses, or organisational difficulties in nurses securing funding and/or study leave to study rehabilitation at post-registration/post-graduate level. Furthermore, professional tribalism, and in some instances turf wars between therapists and nurses for professional dominance in rehabilitation settings, has led to nurses being thwarted from practising to their full scope of competence. Nursing in general is still struggling to identify its specific role within rehabilitation, which can lead to confusion and uncertainty for other professional groups, patients and their families. Nolan *et al.*'s (1997) comprehensive work entitled *New Directions in Rehabilitation* outlined the potential contribution that nurses could make in rehabilitation if they were educated and supported to develop the requisite skills and knowledge. Table 2.1 summarises Nolan *et al.*'s work, detailing the potential roles of nurses in rehabilitation and the necessary skills and knowledge required to fulfil those roles.

Advancing nursing practice in rehabilitation

Advancing nursing practice in rehabilitation is about maximising the scope of one's practice to fulfil the needs of rehabilitation patients within contemporary health service delivery. This invariably means extending and expanding our knowledge, skills and competence underpinned by appropriate theory and evidence. The rationale for this book is advancing nursing practice within rehabilitation. It would therefore seem prudent to define what is meant by advanced practice. Patterson and Haddad (1992) define an advanced nurse practitioner as:

> 'Nurses who will push the known boundaries of their profession, are willing to take the risks and face the challenges associated with breaking new ground and have the ability to articulate their thoughts clearly as they move ahead and develop new nursing knowledge and skills, thus leading their profession forward to meet the needs and demands of society.'

Table 2.1   Potential roles of the nurse. Adapted from Nolan *et al.* (1997).

Role	Knowledge/skills
Assessment of physical condition, delivery of evidence-based care and prevention of secondary complications	• Detailed knowledge of relevant anatomy, physiology and pathophysiology. • Detailed knowledge of contemporary evidence-based treatment modalities and risk management strategies to prevent complications.
Education/counselling	• Detailed knowledge of adult learning and counselling theory. • Ability to assess readiness, capacity and motivation to learn.
Psychosocial interventions	• Knowledge of psychological issues such as altered body image, motivational theories, and clinical depression. • Knowledge of levels and modes of psychological support (see Chapter 4). • Recognising own scope of practice and need to refer patient for more specialist support.
Family carers	• Detailed knowledge of family system theories and ability to assess family dynamics (see Chapter 6).
Coordinating role, liaison and facilitating transition	• Detailed knowledge of multidisciplinary team working, very good communication skills.

The key issues highlighted in this definition are that advancing practice frequently means blurring of traditional professional boundaries, developing new skills and knowledge and developing our role to meet the needs of patients. There is no set repository of skills or knowledge for nurses working at an advanced level, and this is appropriate because it will depend on the type of rehabilitation patient within your caseload, the setting, e.g. community- or hospital-based, and the dynamics of the multidisciplinary team one works within. However, a number of key skills and knowledge are generic to advancing the nursing role, including:

- Holistic health assessment – history taking, physical examination, clinical investigations.
- The informed request and interpretation of clinical investigations.
- Negotiation, management of change and leadership.
- In-depth applied knowledge of relevant anatomy, physiology and pathophysiology.
- Knowledge of appropriate psycho/social theories and their application to the patient group.

- Knowledge of evidence-based practice for the patient group.
- Research skills, both how to interpret research and implement its findings into practice.
- Advanced clinical decision-making and judgements.
- Legal, ethical and professional considerations of advancing the nursing role.
- In-depth understanding of teams and team-working.
- Applied knowledge of how to support and educate informal carers.
- Prescribing of medicines.

    This list is not meant to be exhaustive, but rather a summary of the key skills and knowledge my students and I have needed to advance our practice in recent years. To be able to gain both competence and confidence in the above skills/knowledge, in addition to any specific skills needed for your patient group, it is necessary to undertake a programme of study. This should include both theory and practice, and be flexible enough to meet the needs of practitioners preparing to advance their practice in a variety of settings and with a variety of patient groups. It is important to gain the support and endorsement of your employing organisation and colleagues in the multidisciplinary team: advancing nursing practice cannot be achieved by one individual alone, rather you will become the catalyst to move the service forward. From my own experience of delivering post-graduate programmes to prepare nurses for an advanced practice role, I have found negotiated learning contracts an ideal tool to support the student's learning and role development within their employing organisation. (For further detail on learning contracts please see Chapter 6, and for information on a curriculum to support advancing practice roles please see the concluding chapter.)

    Currently, in the UK, there is no registerable or recordable qualification for an advanced nurse practitioner with the Nursing and Midwifery Council (NMC). To date, a plethora of titles are being used within the UK to indicate that the titleholder is working at a specialist or advanced level, examples include: nurse practitioner, clinical nurse specialist, specialist nurse practitioner, advanced nurse practitioner, nurse consultant, etc. Only one of these titles is recordable with the NMC and that is specialist nurse practitioner. This has led to ambiguity and confusion for patients, their families, other health care professionals and nurses themselves. It is imperative that the public are protected through the professional regulation and registration of nurses working at an advanced level. There now follows a brief discussion of the background to the titles being used by nurses in the UK.

Spheres of professional practice

In the UK, the Scope of Professional Practice produced by the United Kingdom Central Council (UKCC) in 1992 gave practitioners, for the first time, the opportunity to examine and develop their practice according to their patients' needs, and moved away from the concepts of certificated extended and expanded roles. Following this, the UKCC (1994) set out criteria and definitions for four spheres of professional practice:

- Novice
- Primary
- Specialist
- Advanced

The development of specialist and advanced roles is not unique to the UK, indeed over the past 20–30 years in the USA there has been a proliferation of advanced nurse practitioner (ANP) roles. The impetus for the development of the ANP in the USA was to address a national shortage of medical practitioners, particularly within isolated rural communities. Advanced nurse practitioners in the USA are educated to master's degree level and are registered within the state they practice in. They have gained a high degree of professional autonomy including, in many cases, full prescribing rights. Rehabilitation is one of the many specialties that have attracted ANPs. Their roles, although varying from state to state, include advanced holistic health assessment skills, enhanced clinical decision-making and prescription of medication and other treatment options. Like the USA the impetus for the development of specialist/ advanced roles in nursing was due to an anticipated shortage of junior medical staff in the UK resulting from the reduction in junior doctors' hours.

Despite a proliferation of specialist and advanced roles in the UK over the last two decades, the regulation of higher levels of practice has been complex and ambiguous. The UKCC opened a register for specialist practitioners, stipulating that entry to the register would require completion of validated educational programmes to at least first degree level or master's level as well as a minimum of three years post-registration experience within the specific field of practice. Educational preparation for specialist nurse practitioner must comprise equal proportions of practice and theory. However, to date, the professional body have failed to agree on the differentiation between specialist and advanced practice, and subsequently advanced nurse practitioner has not gained registerable or recordable status.

Multifaceted nature of specialist nurses

Specialist nurse practitioners and clinical nurse specialists

The emergence of the Specialist Nurse Practitioner (SNP) Register created a degree of uncertainty for the traditional role of clinical nurse specialist (CNS), which had developed over 20 years in the UK. Since no statutory regulation for the title of clinical nurse specialist exists, this has led to a wide variation in their educational preparation, experience, clinical grading and level of competence. Hamric *et al.* (1996) defined the four sub-roles of a clinical nurse specialist as:

- Expert practitioner
- Researcher
- Educator
- Consultant

The sub-roles defined by Hamric *et al.* appear to be almost identical to the UKCC (1994) definition of a registered specialist nurse practitioner (SNP). It could therefore be argued that there is very little difference between the CNS and SNP roles, except that the latter is protected by professional registration requiring specified educational preparation and a minimum amount of clinical experience within the specialty. This is clearly important to maintain standards of practice, protect the public and enhance the professional standing of nurses taking on additional responsibilities.

By the very nature of their work with a specific group of patients, all nurses working within rehabilitation could be designated as specialists. However, we must be cautious in our differentiation between nurses working within a specialty and registered specialist nurse practitioners. The latter are educated and prepared to work at a higher level in terms of patient assessment, to use diagnostic and clinical reasoning skills and to push the boundaries of practice forward.

Specialist nurse practitioners frequently work autonomously and undertake responsibilities formerly considered to be the domain of medical or therapy professionals. Examples of this include: running nurse practitioner follow-up and review clinics; prescribing medications; requesting and interpreting clinical investigations, such as X-rays; and directly referring patients for various therapies. There are many potential advantages to specialist nurse practitioners taking on these roles, including: reducing waiting lists; freeing up senior medical staff to see more complex cases; offering patients a more holistic consultation; maximising interprofessional working; and providing continuity of care and treatment for patients.

Both clinical nurse specialists and specialist nurse practitioners tend to have no managerial authority over others. Their influence over the quality of patient care comes from clinical leadership, role modelling and the ability to act as change agents. Through the research element of their role, the specialists can influence improvements in practice by both using research as a method of investigating clinical problems and using research-based literature to underpin practice and policy. It is important that those advancing practice through specialist roles remain firmly routed in the ethos of nursing, striving to be 'maxi-nurses' as opposed to 'mini-doctors' (Castledine, 1995).

In the context of informed consent and user involvement in service provision it is imperative that specialist nurses in rehabilitation explain their role and professional background to patients, especially when carrying out procedures that may normally be expected to be carried out by a medical practitioner.

Nurse consultants

In 1999 the Department of Health published *Making a Difference: Strengthening the Nursing, Midwifery and Health Visiting Contribution to Health and Healthcare*. This sets out four levels of practice, as illustrated in Table 2.2. Of particular relevance to this chapter are levels 3 and 4, which define the level of competence,

Table 2.2 Levels of practice for nurse consultants. Reproduced from Department of Health (1999) with permission.

	Typically people will, at a minimum, be competent . . .	Typically posts will include . . .	Typically people here will have been educated and trained to . . .
1	To provide basic and routine personal care and a limited range of clinical interventions routine to the care setting under the supervision of a registered nurse.	Cadets, health care assistants and other clinical support workers.	NVQ levels 1, 2 or 3.
2	To do the above and exercise clinical judgement and assume professional responsibility and accountability for the assessment of health needs, planning, delivery and evaluation of routine and direct care. Direct and supervise the work of support workers and mentor students.	Both newly registered nurses and established registered practitioners in a variety of jobs and specialties in both hospital and community and primary care settings.	Higher education diploma or first degree level, hold professional registration and, in some cases, additional specialist specific professional qualifications.
3	To do the above and assume significant clinical or public health leadership of registered practitioners and others, and/or clinical management and/or specialist care.	Experienced senior registered practitioners in a diverse range of posts, including ward sisters, community nurses and **clinical nurse specialists**.	First or masters degree level, hold professional registration and, in many cases, additional specialist specific professional qualifications.
4	To do the above and provide expert care, to provide clinical or public health leadership and consultancy to senior registered practitioners and others and initiate and lead significant practice, education and service development.	Experienced and expert practitioners holding **nurse consultant posts**.	Masters or doctorate level. Hold professional registration and additional specialist specific professional qualifications commensurate with standards for recognition of a higher level of practice.

experience and educational preparation required for nurses working at nurse specialist or nurse consultant level.

The development of nurse consultant posts was to address the issues of the reduction in junior doctors' hours, and to keep experienced clinical nurses within practice by offering them commensurate salaries and opportunities to develop nursing practice to a higher level. To date, the Department of Health and professional bodies have not stipulated that the nurse consultant title is to be regulated through registration, which may lead to the earlier situation encountered with clinical nurse specialist posts resulting in regional and national variation in terms of experience, qualifications and grade. The Department of Health (1999) specify that nurse consultants will have responsibilities in four main areas: expert practice; professional leadership and consultancy; education and development; and service development linked to research and evaluation. It is specified that nurse consultants must spend at least 50% of their available time in expert clinical practice in contact with patients and clients.

To date, the majority of nurse consultant posts have developed in areas such as critical care, oncology and mental health. However, a small, but significant number of nurse consultants have been appointed within rehabilitation settings. The precise nature and scope of nurse consultants' practice will depend upon local negotiation between the individual, relevant medical consultants and managers, and should be based on patient and service need. From a legal perspective, statute does not stipulate the boundaries between nursing and medical practice except in terms of prescribing. In recent years limited prescribing rights for nurses have been developed in the UK, either through patient group directives, independent or supplementary prescribing.

Nurse prescribing

Since the late 1990s a number of Department of Health directives have aimed to provide nurses with limited prescribing rights. In the first instance this was aimed at district nurses and health visitors who, after educational preparation, were able to prescribe from the formulary for district nurses and health visitors. The formulary mainly comprises a variety of wound dressings, wound cleaning agents and urinary catheters. An extension of independent prescribing was sanctioned by the Department of Health (2003) with the development of the *Nurse Prescribers' Extended Formulary* which covers four main areas of clinical practice: minor ailments; minor injuries; palliative care; and health promotion. The extended formulary includes all general sales list and pharmacy medicines together with a limited list of prescription-only medicines. The items comprising the extended formulary can only be used for treating patients within the four specified areas of practice, and there are a limited number of applications of this formulary. To be eligible to be an independent prescriber using the extended formulary nurses must successfully complete educational preparation comprising 25 days of theory and 12 days of supervised practice with a medical practitioner.

Nurse prescribing is reported to have several benefits, including: saving time for both patients and nurses; being more convenient for patients; and increasing nursing autonomy leading to role satisfaction (Lewis-Evans & Jester, 2004). However, the extended formulary in its present format does not appear to meet the prescribing needs of nurses in advanced roles within rehabilitation. The current alternative is to carry out supplementary prescribing under patient group directives. This allows individual nurses working within advanced roles to administer prescription-only medications such as intra-articular local anaesthetics and steroids, to titrate intrathecal baclofen to control muscle spasm and to titrate first-line drugs used in the treatment of rheumatoid arthritis without having to obtain a medically signed prescription for each individual patient. Patient directives have to be agreed by both the individual health care organisation and the medical team responsible for the patients to be treated under the directive. To fully support nurses in their advanced practice roles it is important for them to be afforded the opportunity to have full prescribing rights dependent on completion of appropriate educational preparation and supervised practice. The current restrictions on independent prescribing rights for nurses working in advanced practice roles may hinder their potential to be autonomous practitioners and provide patients with a high quality seamless service.

Professional autonomy and decision-making

Clearly, advanced nursing roles in rehabilitation require practitioners to exercise high levels of professional autonomy and decision-making. The NHS plan (DH, 2000) sets out a clear agenda to challenge hierarchical ways of working in the NHS with an emphasis on greater flexibility and autonomy for health care professionals such as nurses and therapists. The plan states that nurses and therapists should be afforded greater opportunities for decision-making, specifically in relation to the admission and discharge of patients. Compared to other specialties, rehabilitation has, for a number of years, subscribed to multidisciplinary models of admission and discharge. Clearly, the patient and their family should be at the centre of the decision-making process and play active roles in decisions about issues such as discharge from rehabilitation.

A number of expressions are used to describe the same phenomenon:

- Clinical decision-making
- Clinical judgement
- Clinical inference
- Clinical reasoning
- Diagnostic reasoning

Judgements are reached by assessing the alternatives, while decisions are reached by choosing between alternatives. Decisions comprise both process and outcome, and how we arrive at the decision and the end result are of equal importance. As we advance our practice we must be able to demonstrate a logical and systematic approach to decision-making. Criteria for quality in diagnostic judgements can be either empirical accuracy, or internal consistency and logic. One of the most systematic approaches to clinical decision-making is the hypothetical–deductive approach, also known as 'information processing'. This method embraces two types of reasoning: induction, where data collection leads to the generation of hypotheses; and deduction, where hypotheses are used to predict the presence or absence of data, which clinicians then search for to confirm or deny hypotheses (Higgs & Jones, 1995). This approach comprises four stages:

(1) Cue acquisition
(2) Hypothesis generation (typically 1–3)
(3) Cue interpretation (confirming, refuting or not contributing to the initial hypotheses)
(4) Hypotheses evaluation (weighing up the pros and cons of each possible explanation for your patient's signs and symptoms, choosing the one hypothesis favoured by the majority of evidence)

Harbison (2001) suggested the bias of this approach is 'anchoring', where decision makers tend to continue to favour their initial hypothesis despite incoming contradictory evidence.

An alternative approach to decision-making is using a decision tree or decision analysis to structure the progression of choices and consequences. Some branches represent alternative paths and others possible events. Probabilities for the events are estimated and final outcomes are given values representing patient preference for that outcome. It is a method for rationalising clinicians' behaviour rather than one for explaining how they actually behave (Lilford *et al.*, 1998).

Decision analysis is useful in complex decision-making that does not require an immediate decision. It comprises five stages:

(1) Identify potential choices of action
(2) Assign values (utilities) to each set of possible outcomes (should be based on patient's value judgement using trade-offs or visual analogue scales).
(3) Assign probabilities to chance events (uncertainties) 0 = being impossible and 1 = being certain.
(4) Mathematically combine values and probabilities to establish utilities.
(5) Select the option for action that leads to the highest expected utility.

Traditionally, pattern recognition has been cited as how expert nurses make decisions (Benner *et al.*, 1996), i.e. where a pattern of cues seems to generate outcomes without conscious awareness of the process and is associated with intuition or 'gut feeling'. Buckingham & Adams (2000) suggested that the traditional emphasis on pattern recognition in nursing may be a significant root cause of nurses' weak professional status. However, it is highly probable that, when making complex decisions as you advance your practice, you will need to draw on all these approaches of decision-making, ranging from the intuitive to the purely analytical. Hamm (1988) developed a decision-making continuum theory, which ranges from pure intuition to system-aided judgement and scientific experiment. The most appropriate mode to use for the task in hand depends on three factors:

- The structure of the task
- The number of information cues
- Time available to make the decision

For example, little time, lots of cues and poor structure would lend itself to the intuitive end of the continuum, while lots of time, good structure and few cues would lend itself to analytical modes of decision-making.

An integral part of advancing our nursing practice is to carry out higher levels of decision-making and this contributes to professional autonomy.

Implementing and evaluating advanced nurse practice roles

Developing advanced practice roles requires careful planning and robust evaluation. From an ethical point of view we must ensure beneficence is the key drive to any such development, and ultimately that the advancing role we are providing is improving the quality of care and treatment provided to the patient. Cost-effectiveness must be ensured to avoid the inappropriate use of finite health care resources. Advanced nurse practitioners may provide a service traditionally provided by another health care practitioner, such as a medic. When this is the case it is imperative that the service is as at least equivocal if not improved on what was traditionally provided. It is for these reasons that comprehensive evaluation of advancing nursing practice roles is essential. Evaluation should include:

- Ascertaining patient satisfaction
- Measuring patient outcomes
- Auditing the nature and number of complications
- Reviewing the nature and number of complaints
- Determining the cost-effectiveness of the service
- Auditing waiting times and 'do not attends'
- Establishing the views of other members of the multidisciplinary team on the service

There is a detailed discussion on both the setting up and evaluation of nurse-led services in Chapter 5.

A number of legal issues need to be taken into account, including: professional indemnity; vicarious liability; and informed consent to treatment. It is imperative that your employing organisation is fully aware and consents to you advancing your practice, and that your job description reflects your advancing role. As long as your practice adheres to your employing organisation's policies and procedures and your own job description, then you will be covered in the event of a negligence claim being made. In addition, it is helpful to speak to organisations such as the Royal College of Nursing to check on your indemnity cover as you are advancing your role. In law, as an advanced practitioner, your actions will be judged against the reasonable standard of those normally carrying out the procedure or skill, and this may well mean you are judged against the standard of medical colleagues. This is only right and proper and as professionals we would not expect our practice to be judged at a different level.

Patients must be fully aware of your role and background when consenting to any treatment or procedure, otherwise that consent is not informed. The approach I take to ensure this is: (a) I wear a uniform and identification badge and (b) I introduce myself to each new patient as an advanced nurse practitioner. A frequent question asked by my post-graduate students is: 'What should I say if the patient says "I usually see a doctor"?' This seldom arises, but when it does I always assure patients that following our consultation if either they or I feel there needs to be a second opinion from a medical colleague then this will be arranged.

The literature indicates that one of the most beneficial aspects of advancing nursing practice is improved patient satisfaction. Patient satisfaction is a goal in its own right and there is a direct relationship between satisfaction and concordance with treatment and advice. Conversely, poor patient satisfaction can lead to stress, which has an impact on both physical and psychological well being (see Chapter 5 for further discussion). In addition, the impact of advanced nurse practitioners includes: reducing length of stay; reducing re-admission rates; improving cost-effectiveness; and improving outcomes.

Potential facilitators and barriers to developing advanced practice roles

Jones (2005) conducted a systematic review of studies exploring facilitators and barriers to role development at specialist and advanced level. Although the studies included in the review spanned many specialties, there are a number of commonalities that can be applied to the rehabilitation setting. These relate to the practitioner's personal characteristics and previous experience, professional and educational issues, managerial and organisational issues, relationships with other health care professionals and resources. The factors most frequently identified as important were relationships with key members of the organisation/team, clear role definition and unrealistic expectations of the role. The experience of a significant number of my advanced practice colleagues is that often the organisation does not put in place the necessary support mechanisms for the role, such as administrative support and office space. Also there is a lack of understanding of the role by other members of the multidisciplinary team leading to confusion about responsibility and accountability.

Conclusions

This chapter has attempted to explore the actual and potential role of nurses and nursing within rehabilitation. Clearly, nurses have the potential to make a significant contribution due to the uniqueness of their 24-hour presence; the ability to integrate new skills learnt in therapy are integrated into all aspects of the patient's day, so maximising the time patients spend in meaningful therapeutic activity. Also, nurses have an important role in preventing secondary complications and ensuring that specialist knowledge and skills in pain management, continence promotion and tissue viability are used to optimise the well being of the patient to enable them to actively engage in the rehabilitation process. However, nurses still find it difficult to articulate their specific contribution in rehabilitation compared to other professional groups, such as therapists and medics. Furthermore, the transition from doing things for the patient to a model of maximising patient independence can be a difficult transition. The important factors are (1) that nurses have the appropriate skills and knowledge to prepare them for their potential role in rehabilitation, and (2) that they are empowered to articulate their contribution within the multidisciplinary team by the employing organisations' culture and systems.

Advancing our practice has the potential to make a significant positive impact on patient outcomes and satisfaction and to maximise the role satisfaction of nurses. The development of advancing practice roles requires careful planning and negotiation with other members of the multidisciplinary team to avoid confusion and resentment regarding roles and responsibilities within the team and to have support from the employing organisation in terms of support mechanisms.

References

Benner P., Tanner C. and Chesla C. (1996) *Expertise in Nursing Practice: Caring, Clinical Judgement and Ethics*. New York, Springer.

Buckingham C. and Adams A. (2000) Classifying clinical decision-making: a unifying approach. *Journal of Advanced Nursing*, **32** (4), 981–989.

Castledine G. (1995) The role and criteria of an advanced nurse practitioner. *British Journal of Nursing*, **4** (5), 264–265.

Department of Health (1989) *Caring for People: Community Care in the Next Decade and Beyond*. London, DH.

Department of Health (1998) *The New NHS. Modern and Dependable: A National Framework for Assessing Performance*. London, National Health Service Executive.

Department of Health (1999) *Making a Difference: Strengthening the Nursing, Midwifery and Health Visiting Contribution to Health and Healthcare*. London, DH.

Department of Health (2000) *The NHS Plan: A Plan for Investment: A Plan for Reform*. London, DH.

Department of Health (2003) *Nurse Prescribers' Extended Formulary. Proposals to Extend Range of Prescription Only Medicines*. London, DH.

Ellul J., Watkins C., Ferguson N. and Barer D. (1993) Increasing patient engagement in rehabilitation activities. *Clinical Rehabilitation*, **7**, 297–302.

Hamm R. (1988) Clinical intuition and clinical analysis: Expertise and the cognitive continuum. In: *Professional Judgement: A Reader in Clinical Decision-Making* (J. Dowie and A. Elstein, eds). London, Cambridge, pp. 78–105.

Hamric A., Spross J. and Hanson C. (1996) Surviving system and professional turbulence. *Advanced Nursing Practice: an Integrative Approach*. Philadelphia, W.B. Saunders.

Harbison J. (2001) Clinical decision making in nursing: theoretical perspectives and their relevance to practice. *Journal of Advanced Nursing*, **35** (1), 126–133.

Higgs J. and Jones M. (1995) *Clinical Reasoning in the Health Professions*. Oxford, Butterworth–Heinemann.

Johnson J. (1995) Achieving effective rehabilitation outcomes: does the nurse have a role? *British Journal of Therapy and Rehabilitation*, **2** (3), 113–118.

Jones M. (2005) Role development and effective practice in specialist and advanced practice roles in acute hospital settings: systematic review and meta-synthesis. *Journal of Advanced Nursing*, **49** (2), 191–209.

Lewis-Evans A. and Jester R. (2004) Nurse prescribers' experiences of prescribing. *Journal of Clinical Nursing*, **13** (7), 796–805.

Lilford R., Pauker S., Braunholtz D. and Chard J. (1998) Decision analysis and the implementation of research findings. *British Medical Journal*, **317**, 405–409.

Nolan M., Booth A. and Nolan J. (1997) *New Directions in Rehabilitation: Exploring the Nursing Contribution*. Research Report Series No. 6. London, English National Board for Nursing, Midwifery and Health Visiting (ENB).

Patterson C. and Haddad B. (1992) The advanced nurse practitioner: common attributes. *Canadian Journal of Nursing Administration*, **5** (4), 18–22.

UKCC (1992) *The Scope of Professional Practice*. London, UKCC.

UKCC (1994) *The Future of Professional Practice: The Council's Standards for Education and Practice Following Registration*. London, UKCC.

Waters K. (1996) Rehabilitation: core themes in gerontological nursing. In: *A Textbook of Gerontological Nursing: Perspectives on Practice*. London, Baillière-Tindall, pp. 238–257.

Chapter 3
Rehabilitation Settings

Rebecca Jester

Traditionally, rehabilitation has been delivered mainly within inpatient settings. In recent years, however, there has been a move toward the provision of rehabilitation within community, primary and outpatient settings. The shift in emphasis from hospital to community-based services has been in response to a number of factors, including: the realisation that hospitalisation is not therapeutically beneficial for many, specifically the very young and older people; that rehabilitation is more realistic in the home setting; a shift of power to fund and commission services to primary care; a reduction in the number of hospital beds available; and an increasing demographic population requiring rehabilitation services.

Also, there has been a gradual move away from medically led rehabilitation toward a more holistic approach, with many new services being led by specialist nurses. The specialist rehabilitation nurse has an important role in the assessment of patients and their informal carers to ascertain the optimum rehabilitation setting for them, be that at home or in a specialist inpatient unit. Many specialist nurses working within rehabilitation will find their role involves working across traditional boundaries of community and tertiary settings. This, of course, provides an ideal opportunity to maximise seamless care and provide continuity for the patient and their family. However, it is highly likely that, as specialist nurses in rehabilitation, our roles will become much more focused in the community setting, either directly as members of specialist community-based rehabilitation teams or as a consultant and resource to community teams providing rehabilitation services and ensuring optimal co-operation and collaboration between tertiary and community-based rehabilitation services. The aim of this chapter is to critically evaluate these new ways of working and the inherent shift of knowledge and skills required. Indicative content includes:

- Rehabilitation in the general inpatient setting
- Rehabilitation in a specialist tertiary rehabilitation setting
- Rehabilitation at home/in the community
- Acquisition of skills and knowledge to work across tertiary and community rehabilitation settings

Rehabilitation in the general inpatient setting

There is unequivocal evidence that patient outcomes are better when rehabilitation takes place in a specialist rehabilitation unit rather than the patient remaining in a general inpatient setting (Wade & de Jong, 2000). However, as outlined in Chapter 1 rehabilitation is a goal-directed process and not a physical location. Furthermore, rehabilitation must be begin as soon as the patient is medically stabilised following trauma or disease. This often means the process should begin within a general inpatient setting such as a medical unit following stroke or a trauma unit following hip fracture. Sirois *et al.* (2004) affirm the importance of early transfer from acute units: they reported that shorter administrative delays were associated with shorter rehabilitation length of stay, improved cognitive function and improved motor function at discharge. Rapid transfer of patients to inpatient rehabilitation can affect rehabilitation outcomes positively, and can also lead to an economy of resource use in both acute and rehabilitation settings. However, these factors do not negate the reality that patients frequently have to stay on acute inpatient units while waiting for either a place on a specialist inpatient rehabilitation unit or discharge to home-based rehabilitation services. The specialist rehabilitation nurse has two important functions: providing support and education on the rehabilitation process to nurses and other health care professionals working on an acute unit; and ensuring the effective and timely assessment of patients with regard to their transfer to specialist rehabilitation services.

The need for joined up working between acute and rehabilitation services is paramount to successful outcomes for the patients. We need to consider the following:

- Are there open and clear channels of communication between the acute and rehabilitation teams?
- Are there robust unambiguous criteria for assessing the suitability of patients to transfer to specialist rehabilitation services?
- Do care pathways reflect seamless integration of acute and rehabilitative phases of the patient journey?
- Have staff on the acute units received education, training and ongoing support on the rehabilitation process?
- Are there opportunities for nurses and therapists to rotate between acute and restorative areas to maximise their knowledge and skills in all aspects of the patient's recovery following trauma or disease?

You may find it useful to use the questions above as the focus for a meeting between acute and rehabilitation staff in your organisation. This will provide an opportunity for identifying any deficits in current systems and for developing a collaborative plan of action to maximise seamless working between acute and rehabilitative phases of the patient journey.

There is a fundamental need to minimise length of stay within inpatient settings, because of the well-documented deleterious effects of hospitalisation, specifically for older people. These effects include: the impact of institutionalisation, such as loss of independence, deterioration in cognitive function, rapid disintegration of social networks and depression (Sutherland, 1999; Bennett, 2000). There is a relatively small window of opportunity when patients are ready to be engaged in rehabilitation, if this opportunity is missed patients can quickly become hospitalised resulting in loss of independence and learned helplessness. Therefore, it is imperative that a comprehensive assessment of patients and development of their rehabilitation goals is undertaken as soon as they are medically stabilised.

The specialist nurse must support staff on acute units to actively participate in the assessment and goal planning process with the patient and their family. In addition, there needs to be educational support for acute staff to enable them to gain competence and confidence in specific rehabilitation skills. Several approaches may be adopted to facilitate learning, including: individualised and team learning contracts, which are discussed in further detail later within this chapter; and rotational opportunities for staff between acute and restorative phases of care. The latter also provides an opportunity to break down any barriers/misunderstanding of each other's roles and facilitates collegiate working toward shared aims and goals. Also, rotation will help to facilitate a multi-skilled team who feel confident to support patients through all stages of their journey to recovery, it provides opportunities for continuity for patients and increased job satisfaction for staff as it provides opportunities to 'see patients through' and see them recovered. The specialist nurse should support the educational preparation of acute staff in terms of rehabilitation skills and knowledge. It is important that clinically based learning is linked into the key skills framework. As discussed in Chapter 2 an integral part of the specialist nurse role is the education of staff, patients and informal carers. The Royal College of Nursing have a specific forum for rehabilitation nursing and provide useful literature, conferences and seminars to keep nurses updated on developments in rehabilitation nursing.

Rehabilitation patients on an acute unit do have full access to clinical investigations, such as radiographs, computed tomography (CT) and magnetic resonance imaging (MRI) scans and prompt attention from the full range of medical expertise if secondary complications occur. This can be seen as a potential advantage over some specialist rehabilitation units geographically isolated from the acute hub of the hospital or home-based rehabilitation services. Strategies to overcome these issues will be discussed in further detail later in this chapter.

Rehabilitation in a specialist tertiary rehabilitation setting

The National Service Framework for Older People (DH, 2001) affirmed the importance of specialist rehabilitation units, and stated every general hospital that cares for stroke patients must have introduced a specialist stroke service by 2004. However, a study by the British Association of Stroke Physicians reported that few Trusts had all the components in place for specialist stroke services and availability did not match demand (Rodgers *et al.*, 2003). (For further specific detail on stroke rehabilitation units see Chapter 8.) This situation is not unique to stroke rehabilitation, many NHS organisations continue to struggle to develop and sustain specialist rehabilitation units, either due to insufficient funding or the inability to recruit appropriate staff to the specialty, or a combination of these factors.

Specialist rehabilitation centres have often been situated in relatively small and frequently dilapidated hospital premises that are geographically isolated from the main hub of the organisation, often resulting in difficulty in gaining rapid access to clinical investigations and consultations from specialist medical staff. Although this geographical isolation may appear to have several advantages as the therapeutic milieu may be more tranquil and have better parking for relatives and staff, it perpetuates the philosophical separation of acute and restorative care, rather than affirming the seamless integration of these aspects of the patient's journey to recovery. Specialist nurses have a vital role to play in ensuring that when new hospital projects are being planned that the physical and philosophical integration of rehabilitation and acute care is maximised from the outset. Furthermore, if the rehabilitation specialist unit is to remain geographically isolated in the medium or long term it is imperative that systems are put in place to ensure patients are able to access clinical investigations and consultation with specialist medical staff as quickly as possible.

Rehabilitation provided by specialist units has several advantages over general inpatient units, including: reducing mortality, improved functional outcomes, reduced length of stay and increased patient and informal carer satisfaction. Although there is inconclusive evidence as to why specialist units are more effective, it is likely to be multifactorial, including: improved multidisciplinary working, clear rehabilitation focus, expertise of staff and availability of resources such as gymnasiums and simulated environments. Also, patients will benefit from being with others who are undertaking the same journey as themselves; often, patients can act as positive role models for those earlier in the rehabilitation journey than themselves. People who have successfully completed rehabilitation often can and want to support others with a similar type of disease and/or trauma. One particularly good example of this I have encountered is the 'hopping mad club', a group of amputee patients who came to the rehabilitation unit regularly and would visit patients who had recently undergone amputation. The role of the expert patient has been highlighted in recent government policy, specifically in new ways of working to improve the quality of life for people with chronic long-term conditions. Expert patients and support groups have a vital role to play in supporting patients and their families to come to terms with life-changing trauma and disease. Specialist units often have strong relationships and knowledge of appropriate voluntary organisations, which may not be known to staff in acute units. Further information on the role of the expert patient can be found in Chapter 10.

Justifiably, specialist rehabilitation units must have specific admission criteria to ensure that those patients who will benefit from rehabilitation gain access as rapidly as possible. Specialist nurses have an important role in working with other members of the multidisciplinary team to develop specific admission criteria that engender National Service Framework recommendations and to ensure the appropriate assessment of potential patients against those criteria. Also, they should work with colleagues within the acute setting to ensure that admission criteria and the assessment of patients is understood by all parties, and that the referral process is transparent and efficient to avoid unnecessary delay in transferring suitable patients to specialist rehabilitation services, minimise inappropriate referrals to the rehabilitation unit and maximise the efficiency of rehabilitation services by effective bed utilisation.

Clearly specialist rehabilitation units have many advantages compared to general inpatient centres, but both modes of service delivery necessitate the patient being isolated from their normal home environment and their family. However, there is evidence to suggest that even within specialist rehabilitation units the time patients spend in meaningful therapeutic activity can be as low as 17% of their waking day (Ellul *et al.*, 1993). There is a growing body of evidence and policy supporting a shift away from tertiary rehabilitation centres toward community-based services.

Rehabilitation in the community

The National Service Framework for Older People (DH, 2001) established the need for seamless care and 'joined-up' working between health and social services and between hospital and home care to meet the needs of older people. Hudgell & Gifford (2004) suggested that the two most important aims of intermediate care are prevention of avoidable admission to hospital and supporting early discharge to home from hospital. There have been a multitude of service developments to meet these aims, such as hospital at home (HaH) schemes and, more recently, case management (see Chapter 10). Home-based rehabilitation schemes may be known by a variety of titles, such as 'rehabilitation outreach schemes', 'HaH', 'community rehabilitation teams', etc. However, the principles of these services are similar in that they aim to provide treatment and care in the patient's own home that otherwise would require hospitalisation, and always for a limited period (Shepperd & Illiffe, 1998). (For ease of reading the term 'HaH' will be used to encompass home-based rehabilitation services.)

HaH schemes serve two principal functions: early discharge of patients from hospital into their own environment and prevention of hospital admission. Typically, this involves early discharge following conditions such as stroke or after procedures such as total joint replacement or internal fixation of a hip fracture.

Patients can also be treated at home to avoid hospital admission altogether, for example during an exacerbation of multiple sclerosis or rheumatoid arthritis. It is important to differentiate between the type of service that HaH provides compared to other community and social services. HaH has clearly defined admission and discharge criteria and provides a specific service such as rehabilitation for a limited period. This means that some patients may not be suitable for home rehabilitation either due to their medical status, past medical history or social circumstances.

The issue of patient and carer choice is important. The optimum setting for rehabilitation for individual patients and their families will depend on a number of factors, including: their coping strategies and locus of control; home situation, including formal and informal social networks; and previous experiences of rehabilitation services. Jester (2003) suggested that if choice is removed from patients regarding where their rehabilitation takes place, this can lead to distress and result in the suboptimal achievement of rehabilitation goals. However, in the context of finite resources, managers of rehabilitation services may consider HaH to be the panacea to reduce bed occupancy and to achieve greater throughput. The specialist rehabilitation nurse has an important role in assessing both the patient's and informal carer's suitability for either early discharge to HaH or admission prevention. This requires careful liaison with other services, and frequently, following discharge from HaH, patients will require ongoing lower intensity support from community health and social services.

How does home rehabilitation operate?

Such schemes must have clearly defined admission and discharge criteria to avoid ambiguity about service boundaries with existing community and social services. Most schemes operate seven days per week, typically between early morning and early evening. Seldom do such schemes provide call out during the night, it is for this reason that admission criteria often require patients to have a co-resident informal carer. Home rehabilitation teams often comprise nurses, therapists and support workers, and a degree of multi-skilling is desirable to avoid the cost of multiple visits by various disciplines. Working with confidence and competence across traditional professional boundaries requires careful educational preparation and consideration of issues of vicarious liability and indemnity. Further discussion of educational preparation can be found below.

There are two basic models of home rehabilitation: either outreach from a rehabilitation service based in secondary care or inreach forming an extension of existing community services managed by primary care trusts. Outreach schemes from rehabilitation centres based within secondary care are typically staffed by professionals from the tertiary centre who will have specialist skills and knowledge within a specific area of rehabilitation, e.g. stroke, spinal injuries or orthopaedics. Hospital-based medical consultants retain medical responsibility for the patients. A potential advantage of this model is that if complications arise and the patient requires either re-admission or access to clinical investigations, such as imaging, it is relatively easy to facilitate as the patient remains 'an inpatient'. Also, the outreach team will have a thorough knowledge of the treatment protocols of the tertiary centre and so continuity of treatment will be maintained. Typically, however, outreach staff lack expertise of community working and may find the transaction of their skills and knowledge into the home environment demanding.

Community rehabilitation teams, which comprise an extension of traditional community services, are usually staffed by community nurses and domiciliary therapists, while medical responsibility for the patient is transferred from the hospital-based specialist to the patient's own GP. These staff will have expertise in working within the community setting, but they may not have specialist rehabilitation skills. Also, access to hospital-based clinical investigations and re-admission to the specialist inpatient rehabilitation unit may be difficult for staff who are not employed by the tertiary centre. Both models have their inherent advantages and disadvantages. The potential disadvantages can be minimised by recruiting staff with both community and specialist rehabilitation experience and by induction, education and mentorship processes as discussed below.

Potential advantages and disadvantage of home-based rehabilitation

The potential advantages and disadvantages of rehabilitation in the home setting for patients, informal carers and health care providers are summarised in Tables 3.1–3.3. Evaluations of home-based rehabilitation services indicate that,

Table 3.1 Potential advantages and disadvantages of Hospital at Home (HaH) for the patient.

Advantages	Disadvantages
• Increased patient satisfaction – feeling more secure and in control at home • Rehabilitation more realistic in the home • Better and quicker recovery in terms of achieving rehabilitation goals, due to increased motivation and more one-to-one time with health care professionals • Reduced incidence of hospital acquired infection and other deleterious effects associated with hospitalisation	• Lack of immediate access to the full range of health care professionals • Lack of immediate access to the full range of equipment and investigations • Limited opportunity to meet other patients with similar conditions who can provide positive role modelling and support • Patients with low levels of intrinsic motivation may not actively engage in therapeutic activity unless under high levels of supervision from health care professionals

Table 3.2 Potential advantages and disadvantages of HaH for the informal carer.

Advantages	Disadvantages
• Not having to travel to and from the hospital to visit their relative • Not being separated from their relative • Feeling more in control and an active participant in their relative's rehabilitation process • Possible financial gain through benefits and allowances	• A fairly high degree of responsibility and possible carer strain • Intrusion to home life due to visits of HaH team, presence of equipment and potential adaptations to the home • Possible financial loss if they have to reduce working hours or take unpaid leave

Table 3.3 Potential advantages and disadvantages of HaH for health care professionals/ service providers.

Advantages	Disadvantages
• Reduction in occupied bed days through early discharge to HaH resulting in better throughput through the rehabilitation service • Higher levels of patient satisfaction resulting in fewer complaints • More opportunities for staff, by rotation from inpatient to HaH settings, which may increase job satisfaction and improve retention • Promotes interdisciplinary working and greater professional autonomy	• Not all patients suitable for HaH, necessitating both inpatient service and HaH resources • Initial setting up cost is high including training of staff • Issues of staff safety in the community setting

generally, patients report higher levels of satisfaction, particularly in terms of feeling in control and having more say in their care and treatment (Shepperd & Illiffe, 1998; Jester & Hicks, 2003a). Home-based patients appear to achieve equivocal functional outcomes compared to those remaining within tertiary centres (Richards *et al.*, 1998), but, on balance, home-based modalities appear more cost-effective (Jester & Hicks, 2003b). Most studies evaluating home-based services report that informal carers make significant contributions and experience some degree of burden, which affirms the need for education and support of family carers by health care professionals (see Chapter 6 for further discussion on informal carer support).

Educational preparation and support for home-based rehabilitation

There are a number of salient differences between providing rehabilitation in the inpatient setting and at home, including: personal safety; working across traditional professional boundaries; working alone with limited access to others for advice and support; increased autonomy; legal aspects of entering patients' homes; and limited access to equipment and clinical investigations. Billingham and Boyd (1997) suggested that working in the community differs from working within the inpatient setting, as it usually involves working alone, often unsupervised, with their work hidden from view in the private arena of people's own homes and working with little or no medical direction. Preparing staff to provide evidence-based rehabilitation in the home setting will depend on their previous experience and knowledge, i.e. do they have rehabilitation knowledge which is based on tertiary care or do they have experience of working in the community? To comply with new ways of working, and specifically skills-based commissioning, it is imperative that we start any educational/training programme for community-based rehabilitation services by asking the following key questions:

- What are the collective team skills and knowledge required to provide the community rehabilitation service?
- What type of patients will be accessing the service? Will it be condition-specific, such as stroke or orthopaedic rehabilitation, or more generic?
- What type of skill mix is required, i.e. medical support, registered nurses and therapists, social workers, support workers, administration?
- Will it form an outreach or inreach service?

The information elicited from the questions posed above should form the basis of a compendium of key skills and competencies. It is highly desirable to move toward a transdisciplinary model of working, which engenders multi-skilling, whilst recognising and valuing unique profession-specific contributions.

The next stage in the process is for each member of the team to self-assess against the key skills and competencies by using, for example, a simple 10-cm visual analogue scale ranging from no previous experience or knowledge to fully competent and knowledgeable. Participants should then be supported to identify areas of skills and knowledge deficits. The next stage is to develop a learning plan to address the identified skills/knowledge deficits, this should include specific details of what level of competence is required, the time scale for achievement, modes of learning and the resources required, including contributions by other members of the multidisciplinary team and educational providers as relevant. Also verification of achievement of competence needs to be assessed and recorded, an example of how this might be structured is provided in Tables 3.4 and 3.5.

It is helpful to have both individual and collective learning contracts, which address skills-based commissioning and help to promote a good understanding and appreciation of each team member's role. Based upon my own experiences of providing educational support to outreach teams, most staff recruited from tertiary care backgrounds identify skills/knowledge deficits in areas including: personal safety in the community (see Table 3.6 for key issues), manual

Table 3.4 Example of learning contract for community-based rehabilitation team.

Learning outcome	Action required	By whom	Resources/protocols required	Review date

Signed:

Participant   Clinical facilitator   Educational facilitator   Manager

Date:

Table 3.5 Assessment component of learning contract.

Learning outcome	Assessment details	Date due	Date achieved	Clinical and/or educational facilitator signature

Table 3.6 Principles of managing personal safety in the community setting.

- All staff must undertake personal safety training and updating, which should include non-violent crisis intervention training: recognising potential aggression, de-escalation and breakaway techniques and awareness of environment.
- All staff should have a mobile phone – to summon advice and support quickly.
- Consideration paid to staff uniform – smart and comfortable clothing that doesn't make them easily recognisable as a health care professional, to minimise risk of drug-related crime.
- Comprehensive team policy including: procedure for reporting in to shift coordinator, awareness of what action to be taken if staff do not report in or are not contactable, doubling up for visits when staff feel vulnerable for any reason, reporting of aggression or violence, assessment of the risk of potential aggression based on patient history, social circumstances and locality.
- Good local knowledge of the locality – liaison with police and local community workers.

handling in the patient's home, legal aspects of entry to patients' homes and working with reduced medical supervision/support. Conversely, those recruited from community backgrounds identify knowledge/skill deficits in the following areas: referral systems for efficient re-admission or clinical investigations and evidence-based management for specific conditions/trauma requiring rehabilitation. There are a number of advantages for both individual practitioners and their supporting organisations to using individual and collective learning contracts rather than formal university-based educational programmes.

Learning contracts characteristically have the potential to facilitate both the growth of the individual learner and their sponsoring organisation (the Trust), and as such they form the foundation for continued negotiation between the training facilitator, the individual practitioner, their clinical preceptor and their manager. Learning contracts are mutually binding agreements, which are negotiated between the stakeholders. Learning contracts have been proven to have the following benefits:

- Participants develop critical thinking by having to negotiate their learning needs and make explicit their aims, objectives and development plans.
- Participants' communication and interpersonal relationship skills are enhanced, as learning contracts require them to present and win their argument at the negotiation level.
- Learning contracts promote a sense of ownership and responsibility in participants by encouraging them to take control of their learning.
- Learning contracts ensure that the participant's learning is linked to the overall objectives of the sponsoring organisation.

As educational and training resources are currently limited within the NHS, it is imperative that programmes of learning develop flexible frameworks, embodying negotiated contracts. These will give more consideration to the needs of the sponsoring organisation supporting the participant to develop new skills. Also, it enables the sponsoring organisation to participate in identifying the individual and collective learning goals and resources required to plan more effectively in terms of the participant's release, balanced against organisational needs.

Regardless of previous experience most staff will require training and education regarding multi-skilling to avoid duplicating patient visits. For example, therapists may be required to take blood, administer subcutaneous injections and review medications, while nurses may have to assess gait and range of movements, evidence-based exercise regimens and mobility techniques and to adapt walking aids, etc. The specialist nurse has a key role in supporting community rehabilitation teams during their educational preparation, in liaison with educationalists and the organisation's clinical governance department and in ensuring that issues of vicarious liability and indemnity are addressed when developing evidence-based protocols.

Conclusions

This chapter has attempted to evaluate the various settings in which rehabilitation takes place. It is evident that, as specialist nurses, we have an important role to play in ensuring seamless working between the acute and rehabilitative phases of the patient's journey. With the continued shift away from tertiary rehabilitation toward primary care-led services, it is imperative that practitioners are supported to develop new skills and knowledge in accordance with the key skills framework, and that individual and collective learning contracts can provide a vehicle for educational preparation and training. In an environment that is target- and cost-effectiveness driven, it is important that patients and their families are assessed on an individual basis to ensure that the most appropriate rehabilitation setting is negotiated with them. With the emergence of skills-based commissioning led by primary care trusts (PCTs), rehabilitation teams must ensure that they can provide evidence of the quality and effectiveness of the service they provide, whether they are hospital- or community-based. Furthermore, specialist nurses within rehabilitation will find their roles increasingly spanning tertiary and community services, and that may require transaction of their skills and knowledge across a variety of settings. They have a key role in ensuring that opportunities for staff to rotate between acute and rehabilitation phases are optimised, and that clear and effective referral and communication pathways are established between the tertiary rehabilitation service and the community centre to maximise collaboration and cooperation.

References

Bennett P. (2000) *Introduction to Clinical Psychology*. Buckingham, Open University Press.

Billingham K. and Boyd M. (1997) Developing Clinical Expertise in Community Nursing. In: *Community Health Nursing: Frameworks for Practice* (P. Gastrell and J. Edwards, eds). London, Baillière-Tindall, pp. 233–245.

Department of Health (2001) *National Service Framework for Older People*. London, The Stationery Office.

Ellul J., Watkins C., Ferguson N. and Barer D. (1993) Increasing patient engagement in rehabilitation activities. *Clinical Rehabilitation*, 7, 297–302.

Hudgell A. and Gifford J. (2004) Intermediate care in a primary care trust. *Nursing Standard*, 18 (22), 40–44.

Jester R. (2003) Early discharge to hospital at home: should it be a matter of choice? *Journal of Orthopaedic Nursing*, 7, 64–69.

Jester R. and Hicks C. (2003a) Using cost-effectiveness analysis to compare hospital at home and in-patient interventions. Part 1. *Journal of Clinical Nursing*, 12, 13–19.

Jester R. and Hicks C. (2003b) Using cost-effectiveness analysis to compare hospital at home and in-patient interventions. Part 2. *Journal of Clinical Nursing*, 12, 20–24.

Richards S., Coast J., Gunnell D. and Peters T. (1998) Randomised controlled trial comparing effectiveness and acceptability of an early discharge, hospital at home scheme with acute hospital care. *British Medical Journal*, 316, 1796–1801.

Rodgers H., Dennis M., Cohen D. and Rudd A. (2003) British Association of Stroke Physicians: benchmarking survey of stroke services. *Age and Ageing*, 32, 211–217.

Shepperd S. and Illiffe S. (1998) The effectiveness of hospital at home compared with in-patient care: a systematic review. *Journal of Public Health Medicine*, 20 (3), 344–350.

Sirois M., Lavoie A. and Dionne C. (2004) Impact of transfer delays to rehabilitation in patients with severe trauma. *Archives of Physical Medicine and Rehabilitation*, 85 (2), 184–191.

Sutherland S. (1999) *With Respect to Old Age: Long-Term Care, Rights and Responsibilities. A Report by the Royal Commission on Long-Term Care*. London, The Stationery Office.

Wade D. and de Jong B. (2000) Recent Advances in Rehabilitation. *British Medical Journal*, 320, 1385–1388.

Chapter 4
Psychological Issues in Rehabilitation

Denise Barr

Introduction

As healthy human beings we have expectations about our ability to move, talk, see, smell, hear and generally get by in life. When faced with physical illness, disease or trauma we turn to health professionals to help us 'fix' the problem. Health professionals, in turn, utilise their knowledge of human anatomy and physiology like a 'blueprint', a baseline of 'normality' against which all treatments will be measured. Of course, health care is never that straightforward. Human beings also have psychological, social and spiritual belief and value systems alongside personal experience that blend to form each unique individual. Once past the mechanics of the human body there is no one 'blueprint', no absolute 'normal'. Faced with such complexity and diversity, how can advanced nurse practitioners begin to assess psychological need in a systematic way, and who exactly should meet that need? To address these issues this chapter includes a discussion of the following:

- An overview of psychological theories and their application to practice
- Levels of psychological support and the role of the advanced nurse practitioner and other members of the multidisciplinary team
- Assessment of psychological status
- Body image/altered body image
- Sexuality

The aim of this chapter is to improve competence and confidence in the assessment and delivery of appropriate psychological care for clients and their families. A brief overview of particular aspects of psychology will be offered to underpin the discussion of psychological care itself. The format for discussion will then follow that of the levels of psychological assessment and support offered in *Guidance on Cancer Services: Improving Supportive and Palliative Care for Adults with Cancer* by the National Institute for Clinical Excellence (NICE, 2004; Fig. 4.1). This model offers a simple but effective framework for practice. Although these levels were designed specifically for people with cancer, they

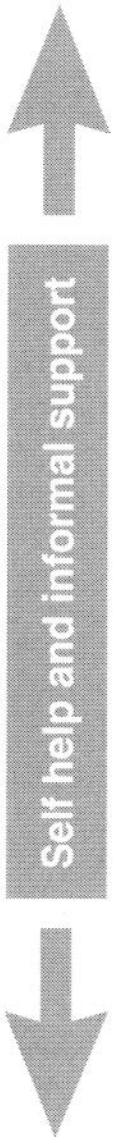

Level	Group	Assessment	Intervention
1	All health and social care professionals	Recognition of psychological needs	Effective information giving, compassionate communication and general psychological support
2	Health and social care professionals with additional expertise	Screening for psychological distress	Psychological techniques such as problem solving
3	Trained and accredited professionals	Assessment for psychological distress and diagnosis of some psychopathology	Counselling and specific psychological interventions such as anxiety management and solution-focused therapy, delivered according to an explicit theoretical framework
4	Mental health specialists	Diagnosis of psychopathology	Specialist psychological and psychiatric interventions such as psychotherapy, including cognitive behavioural therapy (CBT)

(Vertical label at left, with up and down arrows: Self help and informal support)

Fig. 4.1 Recommended model of professional psychological assessment and support. Reproduced from NICE (2004), p. 78.

also offer best practice within the United Kingdom at this present time, and the guidance is therefore seen as applicable and appropriate for any person with health care needs. The term 'he' is used throughout the chapter for ease of reading, but is in no way intended to be sexist. The introduction of the phrase 'and his family' will be taken to mean any person outside of healthcare who is seen as being of great significance to the client.

A brief overview of psychology

The word psychology is derived from the Greek words *psyche* (mind, soul or spirit) and *logos* (discourse or study), i.e. the study of the mind (Gross, 1993).

Within the field of psychology there are different theoretical perspectives on how human thoughts, feelings and behaviours can be affected by a variety of factors and how these factors, in turn, can impact upon the way in which the client and his family deal with ill health. From a nursing perspective a better understanding of these factors can be used to guide not only how we assess psychological need, but also the way in which we offer appropriate interventions.

Social psychology looks at how we make sense of the world around us and how this, in turn, might influence our thoughts, feelings and behaviour. Various theorists, including Freud & Dann (1951) and Bowlby (1969, 1973), have studied child development, aiming to classify human development into stages or processes against which individual progress can be measured. More recently, psychologists Wood *et al.* (2002) have explored the research on development across the lifespan and the changes involved. These changes include moving from milk to solids, learning to walk and to interact with others, starting school, experiencing puberty, leaving school and starting work. There is then independence, marriage with or without children and the process of growing older: developing wrinkles, becoming less able-bodied and therefore more dependent on others. External factors including cultural belief and value systems, socioeconomic conditions and geographical location, alongside internal factors, including biological changes at puberty, add to the complexity of psychological development, as depicted in Fig. 4.2 (Wood *et al.*, 2002; p. 56). These factors are

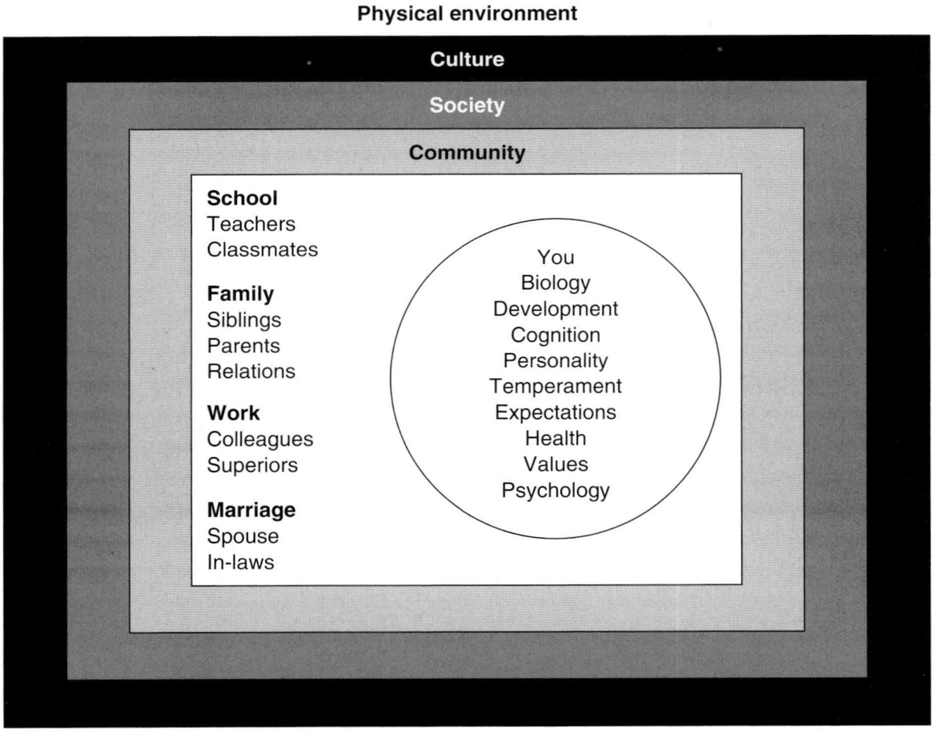

Fig. 4.2 An illustration of contextual influences on the individual. Reproduced from Cooper and Roth (2002), p. 56, with kind permission of Open University Press/McGraw Hill Publishing Company.

so varied that Wood *et al.* (2002) suggested there is no ideal or even normal psychological developmental pathway against which any one person can be assessed. However, this does offer, in very broad terms, a sense of the normal or expected order in which life events should occur. Therefore when an event happens that is seen as being in the 'wrong order', for example a client developing a life-threatening illness whilst his parents are still alive and healthy, we can immediately begin to consider the potentially devastating effect this may have on the client and/or his family.

Scherer (1996) discussed the psychosocial importance of communication, both verbal and non-verbal, in the sending and receiving of strong signals about how others view us, the emotions this evokes and how we can use this feedback mechanism in learning to adapt to changing situations. Of course, many of us now live in geographical areas where the historical culture, belief and value systems are in a state of flux as people move around more with their work. The more cosmopolitan we become the more our social interactions need to accommodate a vast variety of 'social norms', beliefs and values.

Stroebe & Jonas (1996) explained how our attitudes, and therefore behaviours, can be changed by targeted communication on a much larger scale even within a cosmopolitan society. They demonstrated this well by referring to anti-smoking campaigns in Europe, which have led many people not only to stop smoking (behavioural change) but also to regard it as an antisocial behaviour (attitudinal change). Nurses therefore need to assess the individual within the psychosocial context of his life if we are to know where to start in changing attitudes and behaviours that are not helpful to the client and his family.

Alongside developmental and social aspects of what makes us the people we are, there is also the view we have about health and illness. In the nineteenth century the term 'biomedical model' of medicine evolved to guide health care. This model proposed that illness may be caused by a change within normal body function or by external causes, such as bacteria, but that the individual could not be seen as responsible for this and therefore must put his faith in the physician to cure him. The model also proposed that interventions such as surgery or medications were essential in curing the problem, that cancer could cause unhappiness, but not the other way round, and that you were either ill or you were not, there was no grey area (Ogden, 2000). It can be seen that clients who were brought up with this philosophy on health and illness might not feel comfortable challenging a doctor or nurse by offering their own thoughts on 'getting better'.

Throughout the twentieth century this 'biomedical model of care began to be challenged by new ways of looking at health and illness (Ogden, 2000). Engels (1980, cited in Ogden, 2000; p. 5) developed the 'biopsychosocial model of health and illness', which links not only the mind but also the social situation of the client (Fig. 4.3). Within this model the client may be seen as having some responsibility for his ill health, and therefore there is a need to treat the whole person by offering a chance for positive change in the behaviours, beliefs and values that led to the illness. Rather than the ill/healthy choice of the

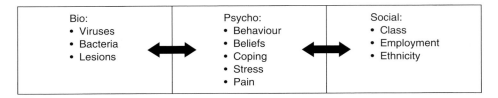

Fig. 4.3 The biopsychosocial model of health and illness. Reproduced from Ogden (2000), p. 5, with kind permission of Open University Press/McGraw Hill Publishing Company.

previous model, this model offers a continuum from ill to healthy along which a client can progress. Clients brought up with this belief system on health and illness may well feel confident in decision-making with doctors, but again assumptions cannot be made.

These two models offer different beliefs on how health professionals should deliver care. As nurses we also have beliefs about clients' care, often describing our practice as 'holistic', caring for the 'whole' client and not just the illness/injury. Woods (1998), however, argued that the term 'holistic care' can be misleading as it does not have one universally accepted definition in nursing. Woods (1998) suggested that there are two main theoretical viewpoints, namely 'strong' and 'weak' holism. 'Strong' involves the thought that the whole is more than the sum of its parts, and therefore reduction to the parts of the whole cannot be seen as holistic, nor can they be understood if considered in isolation. This viewpoint cannot tolerate the idea of specialists within a field of practice, as this would be seen as reductionism. The other 'weak' viewpoint is less radical and recognises the significance of the parts and their impact on the whole. When applied to practice the 'strong' viewpoint is too rigid while the 'weak' viewpoint is more flexible, enabling the 'whole' client to be cared for by a multiprofessional team who together can offer a 'weak', but very effective, holistic approach to care. As an integral member of this team the advanced nurse practitioner will continue to provide a 'reductionalist' aspect of care, which offers a depth and breadth of skills and knowledge in the area of specialism, whilst also offering a holistic approach to psychosocial care, tailored to meet the unique needs of the client.

Clients, as people, may also have strong views on what they perceive to be their own role in health care provision. Rotter (1966) proposed that some people have an internal locus of control, seeing themselves as responsible for what happens to them. Conversely, there are those with an external locus of control who believe that luck, fate, and other people and events are responsible for controlling most aspects of their lives (Rotter, 1966). This certainly seems to 'ring true' in clinical practice. More people than ever seem to be taking an active part in their health care provision, and as the popularity of complementary health care continues to rise, so will the percentage of clients who want to have more information and to take more responsibility for decision-making on care options. All this is a positive move forward; but do our clients have the infrastructure to support them, as this move places considerable onus on the individual at a psychological level and this, in turn, can lead to stress?

From this very broad, basic overview it can be seen that the provision of psychological care can be very complex. Unlike the 'blueprint' of human anatomy and physiology, there really is no such thing as 'normal' when it comes to the psychological self. There are some commonalties, such as the fundamentals of child development and the fact that 'who we are' is influenced by a variety of external and internal factors. Yet each of us is a unique individual requiring care delivery on a humanistic level that celebrates and works alongside that very uniqueness. It is no wonder that it can sometimes take time to truly understand the uniquely complex psychological person who comes to you as a client with a health care need. However, from the outset it is essential to ensure that psychological needs are being met, and this is where the model for psychological care offered by NICE (2004) offers a good framework for practice.

The importance of self-help and informal psychological support

Before discussing the role of health professionals in the provision of psychological care and support, it is important to acknowledge the quintessential role of the client himself and his family in their ability to achieve and maintain optimal psychological well being.

As health professionals we are only invited into the client's life for a finite period, whereas the family are part of that person's everyday life. Therefore the value of support given throughout the illness continuum and beyond by the client's family, his 'informal carers', cannot be underestimated.

Some clients will also choose to take an active role by joining self-help groups and may be involved with these groups long after their initial needs have been met. It is therefore useful to be aware of the well-established self-help groups in your area so that you can offer the client this information.

Informal carers often provide a great deal of valuable support to the client. In an American study exploring support needs it was found that over a quarter of all those asked felt they were heading towards serious psychological problems. However, more of those people sought help from informal sources, such as family and friends, than from any other source (Swindle *et al.*, 2000). Studies such as this highlight the role of carers and the support they must receive in order to continue 'being there' for the client. They also often carry on caring and supporting the client long after the acute intensive input from professionals is over. This vital role is, quite rightly, becoming more recognised and carers' support groups are beginning to emerge. The support for carers is discussed further in Chapter 6 of this book. Throughout all four levels of psychological support discussed in this chapter, the importance of self-help and support by informal sources will continue to be a vital part of the client's recovery.

Levels of assessment and support

Level 1

The guidelines on psychological support at Level 1 (NICE, 2004; see Fig. 4.1) suggest that all staff in contact with clients should be able to offer general emotional care. The assessment at this level involves recognising psychological distress and being competent enough to avoid adding to that distress in any way. The interventions offered include treating clients with dignity, kindness and respect, offering information on available supportive services and having the ability to communicate honestly and compassionately when in consultation with clients and their families (NICE, 2004). Your ability to use communication knowledge and skill adeptly will ensure that you can quickly engage with the client and his family in a respectful and compassionate way. Nurses already practising at advanced level should have all the skills and knowledge to fulfil Level 1 needs with confidence and competence. However, it is worth reviewing these before going onto Level 2.

The key to any assessment is good nurse–client communication. The fundamental aspects of listening and responding, the ability to ask open questions and not feel uncomfortable with short silences and offering unconditional positive regard towards the client, are all vital aspects of good communication skills (Hargie, 1991; Burnard, 1997). Understanding the importance of non-verbal communication skills is also essential. Egan (2001) offers the acronym SOLER as one quick way to check your non-verbal skills when with a client.

> S is for squarely, as in face the client squarely, or as squarely as the situation allows, so the person can see that you are ready to listen.
> O is for open posture, to show the client you are ready to listen.
> L is for lean forward, not too far but just enough for the person to sense that you are interested.
> E is for eye contact, not too intense but sufficient to send a message that you are again interested and want to listen.
> R is for relaxed as this helps the client to also relax and therefore be more able to focus on telling you of their concerns, whilst also helping you to listen more effectively (Egan, 2001).

All these skills are essential, but cannot always be learnt directly from a book. The best way to improve your communication skills is by experiential learning. This can be as simple as getting another person to sit and listen to you for one minute whilst you discuss a hobby or suchlike. You will already have agreed for the person not to speak, but to give you gentle eye contact for the first 30 seconds. Over the next 30 seconds the listener will increasingly look away until they are not looking at you at all. On the many occasions I have used this simple technique to teach the importance of eye contact, it has never failed to highlight how difficult it is to continue talking when the other person looks away too much as the talker stops feeling 'listened to'. There are many excellent communication skills courses around where you learn by taking part in role-play, etc. I would encourage anyone to take part in these, as you are able to practise different ways of approaching a topic or dealing with a potentially distressing situation in the safety of the classroom, therefore not causing distress to a real client whilst you are in the process of learning.

Alongside good communication skills is the need to have some understanding of the degree of adjustment needed in order for the client and family to try and cope with the problem facing them. Brennan (2001) has offered an excellent paper on adjusting to cancer, exploring the personal transition clients make. Although discussed in relation to cancer, the points made with regard to the personal transition clients make are actually just as relevant for any other health-related problem, and it is therefore offered as an excellent read. He suggests that, 'as a result of their social development, people acquire an enormous complex matrix of assumptions about how the world functions, a cognitive map which is being continuously revised' (Brennan, 2001; p. 8). A simple but very useful model on adjustment is also offered (Fig. 4.4).

Within the model there is predictability, based on our matrix of assumptions. For example, if I expect to get from point A to point B within 30 minutes by car to attend a meeting and I do indeed manage this, then my assumption is confirmed. If, however, on the way to point B the car breaks down, I may at first try to restart it then sit for a little while before trying again, assuring myself it will work next time I turn the key (denial). This denial may be okay as the car may well start next time and off I go, reaching the meeting a little later than planned. However, if the car does not start on the second or third time of trying I will begin to get stressed. I will need to take other measures to get the car going again and get to point B. Eventually the mechanic comes and I get to point B much later and very stressed, the meeting is nearly over and that stresses me even more. My assumption about the journey time was not

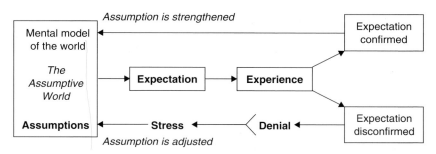

Fig. 4.4   The social-cognitive transition model of adjustment. Reproduced from Brennan (2001), p. 8, with kind permission of John Wiley & Sons.

confirmed. Next time I may well set off earlier (reduce stress) and ensure my mobile phone is working so that I can let people know I will be late (reduce stress). In this way my assumption has been adjusted to take these variables into account: my cognitive map has been revised. This, of course, is a very simple example of how the model works.

Now apply it to a situation within your own sphere of practice, where a client has been given bad news and needs to find ways to adjust. The model can now help you to better understand where the client or carer is coming from. It may be that denial is the right approach for some people some of the time, it may reduce stress for a while. For some people the ability to change their assumptive world to meet new developments may be easy, whilst for others they keep having expectations disconfirmed without actually managing to get out of that loop of thinking. Remember also that the 'expectation confirmed loop' may be a negative or a positive, for example a person may feel they cannot move a joint properly following a trauma because it will hurt, they try and their assumption is confirmed. Over time, the trauma heals but they continue to immobilise the joint for fear of further pain. Eventually the joint will become stiff and painful, reaffirming the belief and requiring professional help to put right the problem. I am sure all of us can recall clients who fit this kind of description. Again, using the model to understand where they 'may be' helps you to better understand their world and therefore, hopefully, take the most appropriate steps to help the situation.

Although initially Level 1 support may appear simple, it can now be seen that we all use extremely complex knowledge and skills each time we interact with our clients and their carers. The ability to be respectful, to communicate in an appropriate way so as not to cause or increase distress will involve ensuring the environment in which you meet is appropriate, that you give time for the client to tell his story and are able to respond appropriately to the situation.

If faced with distress, take time to find out why, it may be that they are adjusting and this takes time. It may be that you need to refer on to someone else who can be more helpful than you for that particular problem. It may be that the client and/or carer already has concurrent psychological or psychiatric needs and that these are being addressed by the relevant professionals. You can liaise with these others as appropriate.

It is not essential to have all the answers the first time you meet a client or to feel you have to immediately 'fix it' if faced with their distress due to inappropriate communication from another health professional. If they leave you feeling they can trust you, that you have given them some ideas of how to proceed, and if they feel they can return to see you again if needed then you have fulfilled the support needs for Level 1. Furthermore, the guidelines suggest that the ability to provide appropriate interventions at Level 1 may prevent the development of more severe problems, thereby affecting demand for services at Level 2 and beyond (NICE, 2004; p. 79). If so, it is a win–win situation for all concerned. However, for those requiring further support and psychological care we will now discuss Level 2.

Level 2

The guidelines on psychological support, at Level 2 (NICE, 2004; see Fig. 4.1), suggest that 'professionals operating at this level should be able to screen for psychological distress at key points in the patient pathway' (NICE, 2004; p. 79). These key points are suggested as being at diagnosis, during treatment, as treatment finishes and at the time of recurrence of the cancer. Again these can be easily changed to other illness trajectories as all have a start point when the diagnosis is made, acute treatment and end of acute treatment phase and, hopefully not too often, setbacks in progress. The extra interventions expected at Level 2 are the ability to offer techniques, such as skilled communication, in helping clients to identify and then solve problems for themselves, alongside the use of screening tools to identify when a situation is beyond your ability and needs referring on to a psychologist or psychiatrist (NICE, 2004).

Within this level the client would need to consent to completing a psychological screening tool, having had it explained to them in terms of its use to monitor how they are adjusting to their situation, who will have access to the answers they give and what will happen if it is felt the client needs specialist help beyond your scope of practice. You therefore need to be aware of the availability and referral procedure for clinical psychology or psychiatry within your health care setting. In clinical practice we have probably all met clients and carers who have shown consternation at the thought of involving a psychologist or psychiatrist to look at their psychological well being. The stigma of needing mental health care remains a concern for most people. Health psychologists are often described as 'people who assess and treat people in distress' (Ogden, 2000). This is a helpful phrase to use when explaining their role or that of the psychiatrist to the client. You can then go on to explain that many people have trouble adjusting to changes in their lives and that they should be offered specialist care, just as they have accepted specialist care for the physical problems they are now experiencing.

There are various ways of screening for psychological distress, including interviewing clients and/or asking them to complete psychological or quality-of-life questionnaires using scoring systems. The distress thermometer (Zabora, 1998; Fig. 4.5) is a simple tool, developed for use by people with cancer. The client rates their distress related to the various problems on an adjacent trigger list as a score from 1 to 10. The Hospital Anxiety and Depression Scale (HADS) was developed by Zigmond & Snaith (1983) originally for use in a medical outpatients clinic to assess anxiety and depression for that particular population of patients, but it has since become widely known and used with other client groups (Snaith, 2003). The Functional Assessment of Chronic Illness Therapy (FACIT) offers a quality-of-life measure that has been adapted and tested for reliability and validity when used in a variety of site-specific cancer and neurological settings, as well as within the general population (FACIT, 2005).

These are just three examples of screening scales that offer a baseline which can then be repeated to monitor the effectiveness of interventions. However,

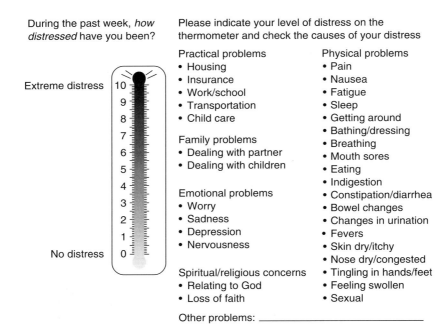

During the past week, *how distressed* have you been?

Please indicate your level of distress on the thermometer and check the causes of your distress

Extreme distress   10

9
8
7
6
5
4
3
2
1

No distress   0

Practical problems
• Housing
• Insurance
• Work/school
• Transportation
• Child care

Family problems
• Dealing with partner
• Dealing with children

Emotional problems
• Worry
• Sadness
• Depression
• Nervousness

Spiritual/religious concerns
• Relating to God
• Loss of faith

Physical problems
• Pain
• Nausea
• Fatigue
• Sleep
• Getting around
• Bathing/dressing
• Breathing
• Mouth sores
• Eating
• Indigestion
• Constipation/diarrhea
• Bowel changes
• Changes in urination
• Fevers
• Skin dry/itchy
• Nose dry/congested
• Tingling in hands/feet
• Feeling swollen
• Sexual

Other problems: _____

Fig. 4.5 The distress thermometer. Reproduced from Foley and Gelband (2001) with kind permission of the National Academies Press.

your local psychological and psychiatric teams may well advocate a particular screening tool not mentioned here. Whichever one is used, please ensure it has proven reliability and validity when used within your client group if it is to guide your practice in knowing when you can continue helping the client yourself and when to refer on for specialist help.

Many clients you meet will not require referral to a psychologist or psychiatrist, but will require help to adjust to the changes that have taken place in their lives due to the illness, disease or trauma. Some people might, at this juncture, begin to consider the need for counselling skills. But what exactly does 'counselling' involve and is this what you are actually going to offer your client? Burnard (2005) has offered a variety of definitions of counselling, ranging from those that offer a way to help another person clarify problems and ways to move forward through to the approach taken by a qualified psychotherapist. Throughout all those definitions there is one-to-one communication, after which the client takes action to help himself. In reality the client may well offer problems that would benefit from the inclusion of other professionals, such as a social worker, occupational therapist, physiotherapist or religious advisor. Therefore it may be more useful to consider our interactions with clients, in terms of utilising advanced communication skills to assess and clarify the problems and decide upon the most appropriate way forward. Although this may involve only one other health care professional, it often involves the combined effort of a multidisciplinary team approach to rehabilitation. The

The Skilled Helper Model

Stage I: What's going on?	Stage II: What solutions make sense for me?	Stage III: How do I get what I need or want?
Story	Possibilities	Possible strategies
Blind spots	Change agenda	Best fit
Leverage	Commitment	Plan

How do I make it happen?

Fig. 4.6 The helping model showing interactive stages and steps. Reproduced from Egan (2001), p. 32, with kind permission of Thomson Learning Inc.

use of some kind of systematic approach to aid communication would ensure that the client and health professionals do not end up talking themselves round in circles without finding ways of improving the client's situation. A variety of approaches or models of helpful communication exist. However, within this chapter, I will give a brief overview of just one model as an example and then encourage you to read further on the topic.

Egan (2001; Fig. 4.6) offered a model of the interactive stages and steps in his model of helpful communication. This model offers a framework for practice, guiding the helper along a pathway that should help the client to tell their story and, in so doing, highlight those 'blind spots' that the client cannot see clearly but which are there and are open to positive change or 'leverage'. The helper then encourages the client to explore the areas open to change, looking for realistic, sustainable goals that the client can commit to. This then leads to discussion on the range of options open to the client that can achieve the agreed goals. After finding the options offering the 'best fit' the client can then, guided by the helper, begin to plan a strategy to achieve these goals (Egan, 2001). Although this may sound a simple model to follow, the skills needed to guide the client through this process should not be underestimated. Anyone who is not skilled in this kind of advanced communication should attend an experiential learning course on advanced communication skills. There you will be able to practise skills with other professionals in the safety of the classroom before using them in clinical practice. This will allow you the time to explore ways of phrasing questions, to practise your non-verbal skills and to receive feedback aimed at improving your competence and confidence. For those who already practise this kind of advanced helpful communication, the use of clinical supervision offers an ongoing way to 'touch base' with someone more skilled than you are. This will offer you support whilst also keeping your practice reflective, enabling you to learn and fine-tune your skills still further. Whatever your starting point and choice of framework/model/ approach to helpful communication, your skills need to be kept updated and reviewed regularly to ensure you always offer optimal service to the benefit of your client.

It may be that by telling their story the client or carer highlights their lack of knowledge of service provision, which for some reason was not offered at Level 1 or was offered but not remembered due to the stress of the initial situation. This information need can then be addressed.

Within the model offered by Egan (2001) there are the 'possibilities' and 'possible strategy' steps. This is where the helper can introduce the idea of utilising the skills of the multiprofessional team to help the client realise their goals. It may be that financial concerns merit the introduction of a social worker or an occupational therapist (OT) to carry out an assessment at work or home and then provide equipment aimed at meeting the client's needs, or the client may have spiritual concerns that could be helped by talking further with yourself or with a chaplain or other religious advisor. Remember, spirituality and religion are not synonymous. Spirituality centres around questions such as, 'why am I here?', 'why me?', 'what does all this really mean?' and does not have to find an answer in a religious way. Religion offers a set of beliefs and values that, for some people, may be able to answer these spiritual questions and offer a sense of calm or inner strength. This is why for those people who do not have a religious belief the chaplain may not always be the best person with whom to discuss spirituality.

There may well be a point in the conversation when it is obvious to you that the client is nursing a big fear about, for example, the disease trajectory. For some, just saying their fear out loud can, in itself, be therapeutic. If you get that feeling then do ensure you encourage them by probing gently. Again, if this technique is new to you do practise it first by using role play with col-leagues and trying out dialogue, such as: 'Sometimes we find it hard to talk about the things that frighten us most, yet people say that once they say the fear out loud it starts to get smaller. If ever you feel like that I am here and will listen.' The art is in offering to listen without making the client feel in any way weak for having their fear, and in being confident enough to leave that thought with them and see if they follow it through. Remember also that the client may choose never to tell you, but to share this fear with another professional or with a friend or carer. The important part is the bit where you acknowledge that it's okay to have fears, as this enables the client to say theirs out loud to the person they do see as the most appropriate person.

Another area of concern for many clients in rehabilitation is one of body image changes due to the disease/illness/trauma. Helpful communication skills will enable you to elicit these concerns, whilst an understanding of body image will help to guide goal setting with the client.

Altered body image

Schilder (1935; p. 17) defined body image as 'the picture of our body which we form in our mind, that is to say the way in which our body appears to ourselves'. This is a good starting point as it focuses on the unique way we all see ourselves. We place different values on the various parts of our body, depending on their importance to ourselves. Ask a group of colleagues to pretend they have to insure one part of their bodies for more than any other part, then ask which part they each choose and why. Some may choose their sight or their hearing, whilst others may choose their face, legs or arms. In a teaching session on body image recently one student chose her pubic hair, without which she would have felt ugly and less sexual. The others were initially embarrassed by this answer, but it led into a conversation about sexuality and the need to enable people to express their concerns without allowing your own personal views to get in the way. Others in the group then said that they had thought about sexual organs but did not want to appear silly or self-obsessed by saying these parts. We all agreed that what others think of you is also important. Professionally, this may prevent the client from telling you their real concern for fear that you will either think less of them or not take their concern seriously, because they think you do not see it as being so important. The point is that, as with all other things in life, you cannot assume anything when it comes to body image. You need to ask, using all your advanced communication skills to ensure you do not block the client the minute they move into territory you feel uncomfortable in. Remember also that you are not the only health professional caring for the client. If you do not feel comfortable with their concern, then acknowledge that you have listened by clarifying their problem and then suggesting that you do not know enough about this to help them but can find someone who will be able to help. Remember that knowing the limits of your knowledge and ability is a true strength, as it ensures the most appropriate person always offers the client the most appropriate care.

As with helpful communications, there are models of body image care that can be used as frameworks for practice. Within this chapter the model offered will be that by Price (1990a), although, again, the advice would be to read further into the topic and decide which one you and your colleagues feel to be the best fit for your client group. One useful read might be the handbook on body image theory, research and clinical practice by Cash and Pruzinsky (2002).

Price (1990a) identifies dimensions of body image (perception, cognition, social and aesthetic) and proposes a five-concept body image model. These concepts are: body reality (the body as it really is); body ideal (beliefs about how the

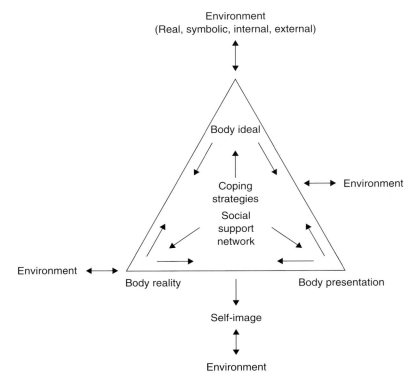

Fig. 4.7   The body-image care model. Arrows indicate direction of influence of interaction. Reproduced from Price (1990a), with kind permission of *Journal of Advanced Nursing*.

body should be); body presentation (how the body is presented to the outside world); and two mitigating personal responses: coping strategies and social support networks. The three body concepts are placed at the three corners of a triangle, with the strategies helping to keep it equilateral to maintain 'balance' and within which the individual has an acceptable body image (Price, 1990; Fig. 4.7). At face value this seems simple, keep the sides of the triangle equal and all will be well. Of course it is not so easy in practice. It may be that the person has poor coping skills or no social network. It may be that the person has alopecia, in which case a wig will help with body presentation, but what about eyebrows and eyelashes? Some people need to take medication to maintain optimal health, which affects body reality by causing a noticeable weight gain. Remember also that many of us have an acceptable timeline for body image – with the young expected to be supple, smooth-skinned, agile people – whilst older people develop wrinkles and arthritis. What then of the young person who develops arthritis or the pensioner who opts for cosmetic surgery to stay young looking? One person may see a urinary catheter as helpful, whilst another person of the same age sees it as a total invasion of their body space. What the model does offer is a framework for assessment, enabling you to find out just how big the gap is between the ideal and the reality for the individual client and what body presentation can do to help regain some balance.

Price (1990b) then offers his model without the triangle but within the framework of multiprofessional working in the rehabilitation setting (Fig. 4.8). The complexity of the problem is broken down and offers a good starting point for deciding not only what is needed, but also who may be the best person, or people, to offer it. To test this model in practice let us take fictitious Mr X, age 48, who lost his right arm in a road traffic accident three weeks ago. The driver of the other vehicle has been charged with dangerous driving and the case is in the hands of the insurance companies. Mr X is happily married with two teenage sons and a six-year-old daughter. He worked as a car mechanic before his accident. His hobbies are golf and 'drinking with the boys'. He is well known locally and likes to help out in the community. You are the advanced nurse practitioner who is to be involved in his rehabilitation, but you were on annual leave when his accident happened. On your return to work, staff voice concern that he is due to be discharged from hospital any day now but is still not able to look at the stump or take any part in caring for it.

Using the triangular model (Price 1990a) we can start to consider questions with regard to social support: How is his wife coping? How have his friends responded? How does he feel about their reaction to his situation? Has Mr X had to cope with stressful situations before and, if so, what coping strategies did he use and how did they help? What, if anything has yet been said about the future for his job, is his boss offering support financially? Does Mr X have religious beliefs and attend his place of worship regularly, if so does this help him at all? Has he spoken about the driver of the other vehicle, and if so what has he said? What is his score on your psychological screening tool? Then onto the body image itself. How does the loss of an arm affect his view of his body image, does it destroy any hope of ever reaching his perceived body ideal, will a prosthesis be seen as a help or a hindrance? How big is the gap between his body reality and ideal? Has this changed in the last week? How much adjustment is needed in other parts of his life to make this change in body image more acceptable and to enable him to get back to some kind of 'ordinary' life?

Just thinking of the questions can open so many areas for potential concern, that how will you start to help by asking these questions without overwhelming Mr X. This leads to Fig. 4.8. Take a look at all the people who can be involved. A team approach is the best way forward. Mr X and his wife will be the central members of this team. Acknowledging the problem with Mr and Mrs X and the need to all work together as a team to help will be the first step. The assessment can then begin. You will have all your questions, but, again going back to a model for helpful communication, many of these may well be offered by Mr X and his wife as part of telling you their story, avoiding the need for you to simply work your way through your questions. Also, by following Mr X's agenda you may also recognise some 'black-spots' open to 'leverage'. Once the story is told you can then probe gently around the three

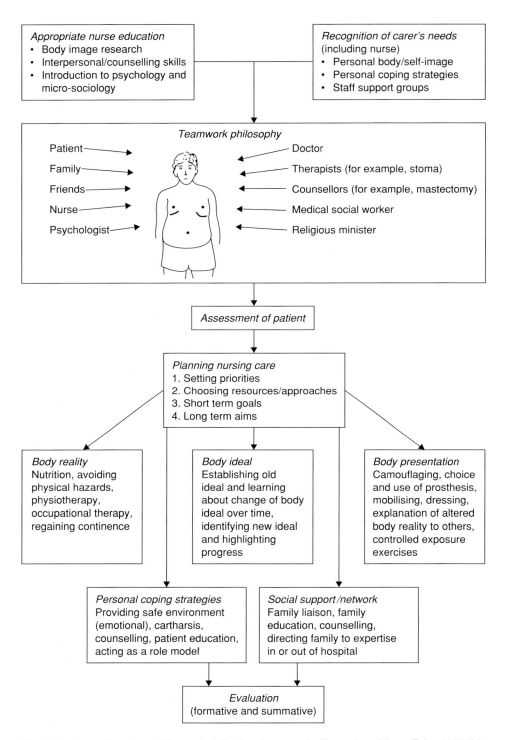

Fig. 4.8 Care planning within a rehabilitation framework. Reproduced from Price (1990b), p. 82.

areas of body reality, ideal and presentation and the impact of coping and social concepts upon these.

Following the assessment it transpires that Mr X is usually a happy man, with a ready smile, quick to find the funny side of sad situations as a way of coping. However, although he is still trying to use this strategy, it is not working as the problem is much bigger than anything he has ever had to deal with before. His boss is supportive, but accepts that there may not be a suitable job for Mr X to return to. Mrs X has not worked since the children were born. Although she is willing to find work, she is nervous and Mr X feels this changes his role within the family as the breadwinner. He cannot see a way to play golf with only one arm and will not be able to hug his children. This then leads him on to expressing concerns at how his body looks now, and he makes a joke about his wife not wanting a one-armed man. Although joking, the anxiety is clear in his voice and his wife's eyes lower. Maybe she is not sure if she can cope with the change. It may be that the couple are experiencing changes in their sexual relationship, or that Mr X feels less of a man, with all the changes in his role as breadwinner and provider, and that this, in turn, is affecting his own sexuality thereby causing conflict between them.

These topics of sexual intimacy and sexuality are very sensitive. I remember a colleague recalling a study day he had been to on helping clients explore these concerns. For the 'icebreaker' the participants had been asked to get into pairs and discuss their last sexual experience in detail. Everyone sat in stunned silence. The lecturer had made her point. None of them felt able to disclose this kind of intimate information to a stranger, just as our clients and spouses cannot necessarily be expected to sit down and discuss their sex life or changes in perception of their sexuality openly 'just like that' on the first meeting or even on the first few meetings. In the case of Mr X and his wife it is enough to just say 'some people in your situation have expressed concerns about how the change in appearance might affect their own sexuality, feelings towards each other and their intimate relationship. If either of you have these kind of concerns I am here to listen'. This should let them know you will not shy away from this kind of concern. It also acknowledges that either of them may have concerns and can feel confident enough to voice these, either now or at a later date if they need to.

Of course, there is always the possibility of 'opening a can of worms', whereby one of the couple will open up whilst the other one shows upset or anger at this disclosure. This is where all your communication skills come into play, for you will need to find a way to acknowledge the concerns of the one whilst also being aware of the feelings of the other. In some cases the act of voicing concerns will be therapeutic in itself, as the partner may be able to offer support and encouragement. In other cases the body image framework can be used to assess and plan appropriate care. If the problem is obviously bigger than your ability to deal with it, then say so and offer to refer on to the appropriate professional in a timely manner before their situation gets any worse.

Having completed an initial assessment you need to clarify Mr and Mrs X's concerns. Then you need to discuss an order of priority with the couple, utilising your past knowledge and experience in guiding them towards realistic short-, medium- and then long-term goals that will involve other professionals all being kept up to date. Acknowledge where the gaps between ideal and reality are widest and the need for time to adjust and look for compromise between what is wanted and what is possible. This way you will not create an expectation that cannot be met since your relationship is built on honesty and trust. The multiprofessional team can then work toward these goals together with Mr and Mrs X, evaluating and reassessing as needed to ensure optimal care at all times.

The use of a model for helpful communication offers the professional a flexible framework that can be adjusted to meet the unique needs of the individual. Using it not as 'counselling' but as 'helpful communication' facilitates the introduction of other professionals and carers into the framework to the benefit of the client in a way that 'counselling' may be unable to offer. Adding in a model for body image care can further enhance care delivery by enabling you to better understand the complexity of the issues for the client, and then to explore ways to help them improve their psychological well being. Once again, remember that the psychologist should be seen as an extended member of your team if not an actual team member, and that the screening tool should indicate when referral is needed. Level 2 psychological care requires the addition of an advanced level of skill and knowledge in advanced communication, models for body image care and use of appropriate screening tools.

These come into even sharper focus when the client's health does not improve and the focus of care moves from 'cure' to palliation. Field and Copp (1999) suggest that sensitive open communication, at a pace the patient is ready to receive it, usually leads to less anxiety for all concerned, facilitates the ability to offer palliative care options and to stop unnecessary treatments. From their observational research, Glaser and Strauss (1965) described instances where some hospital staff felt able to communicate openly with dying patients whilst others either kept patients ignorant of their impending death or both parties had chosen not to acknowledge the fact by pretending all was well.

A study by Gott *et al.*, (2001) showed there was low concurrence between nurses and doctors in an acute hospital setting as to when patients were 'palliative'. Other studies found that nurses and doctors would often overestimate the life expectancy of dying patients (Parkes, 1972; Heyse-Moore & Johnson-Bell, 1987; Buchan, 1995; Viganò *et al.*, 1999). Evans & McCarthy (1985) suggested that some doctors may need to maintain the uncertainty of disease outcome, either to justify continuing active treatment whilst the patient is dying or to avoid the patient feeling rejected. Christakis (1998) suggested that the physician may see the uncertainty as a dilemma, not wanting to refer to palliative care services too early, which then leads to late referral.

Doyle (1999) proposed that some staff, having been on a short palliative care course, may consider themselves able to deal with any situation without specialist support. These problems ring true in clinical practice and often lead to patients only being referred to palliative care teams hours or a day or two before death when the family is in crisis. Effective communication is pivotal in reducing tensions and ensuring the patient's symptoms are controlled and the patient's and family needs are acknowledged and met. Earlier identification of the impending death and appropriate proactive management would avoid the majority of the crisis situations for patients, their families and staff, and increase patient and informal carer satisfaction with service provision. Gott *et al.* (2001) recommended further education for doctors and nurses working in acute hospitals on how to best utilise specialist hospital palliative care services.

If you have taken the time to lay down a firm foundation of trust and respect within your professional relationship, not only with the client and family but also with your local palliative care team if there is one, then you should not find yourself in a dilemma. The change from curative to palliative care should have been slowly happening: maybe introducing the palliative care team for symptom control advice or added support in the first place, then slowly increasing their input as that of the acute team remains but is less prominent. In this way the patient will, hopefully, not feel 'abandoned' by you. Without a local palliative care team you will need to ensure that the client and family understand the change in gear from curative to supportive care. You must not give false hope or expectation, or they will stop trusting you. If the patient is new to you then your first step is to find out how the patient and family have taken the news of the poor prognosis and their concerns at this time.

We cannot appreciate the suffering that clients and their families may go through at this time, when the only future certainty is death of the patient. How will they cope? Can they find any sense of hope in this situation? MacAdam & Smith (1987) suggested that because suffering is unique to the individual it can only be judged by the person experiencing it within the context of their expectations, hopes, fears, philosophies and beliefs. This is a useful definition, as it begins to build a picture of just how complex suffering can be and how coping and hoping are woven into it. In Egan's opinion (2001), helping another person starts by listening to their view of the situation. This is certainly relevant when trying to help a patient or family member hope and cope, since one must first help them to identify any aspects of suffering open to positive change.

Keep listening to the client and family, be responsive to their needs and, again, remember that you do not have to be a specialist palliative care nurse yourself. The multiprofessional team can expand to include the palliative care specialists needed to focus care on optimal quality of life and dignity up to the very last moment of the client's life, and then go on to support the family in their bereavement.

Levels 3 and 4

Levels 3 and 4 of the supportive care guidelines are to be carried out by appropriately trained professionals, namely psychologists and psychiatrists (NICE, 2004; Fig. 4.1). For the advanced nurse practitioner the most important thing to remember about these levels of care is that they exist. Ensure you have effective screening tools in place. There should be no delay in referral, as this would put the client at risk of seriously delaying their return to psychological well being.

The care you are providing will not necessarily change. The use of a psychologist or psychiatrist is often 'as well as' not 'instead of' your care, as again this professional will simply become an extended member of your team whilst involved in care delivery to the client and/or family.

Looking after yourself

Optimal psychological care can be a complicated and time-consuming business. Maybe instead of using the troublesome term 'holistic care' we should rename this approach 'humanistic care', where we respect and value our fellow man with the beliefs, values and life experiences that blend together to make him the unique individual he is. This very uniqueness is then acknowledged, enabling the needs of the client and family to be addressed in a partnership **with** him and not **for** him.

Yet this 'connecting' with clients on a humanistic level brings with it the need to ensure you are supported sufficiently to continue offering support to others. Clinical supervision is an excellent way to ensure support whilst also challenging you to reflect and learn for the future. Ensure you take time to be kind to yourself and always aim for a fine balance between home and private life. Years ago a social worker showed me a simple way to maintain balance in life. Draw a circle. Label all the things you do for others with an arrow pointing out of the circle. These things may include supporting colleagues and clients at work, caring for family members, offering support to friends, helping out at church, etc. Then draw arrows pointing inwards and label these with the things you get back. These may be the love of your family, time to yourself at the gym, support from colleagues, etc. As long as the arrows going in are about equal to those going out you should be okay. However, once the outward arrows far outweigh the inward arrows you are giving much more than you are receiving and this will not be sustainable over time, you need to take steps to redress the balance. Find out more about your local psychology service. Do they offer staff support? If so, then this can be an excellent way to take time to rebalance your life, perhaps by improving coping skills or using their specialist counselling skills to help find areas of your life open to positive change. Of course, you may have more arrows going in than out, if so you are truly blessed with the ability to look after yourself.

Conclusions

There is an increasing need for advanced nurse practitioners to ensure they possess advanced communication skills and knowledge as an integral part of psychological care. The aim of this chapter was to improve competence and confidence in the assessment and delivery of appropriate psychological care for clients and their families. The use of the levels of care offered within the NICE guidelines (NICE, 2004) has offered us a framework for discussion. It can been seen that these levels of care are appropriate for any client with health care problems, and are appropriate from the time the client first requires health care until they fully recover or die.

As advanced nurse practitioners you will often be working at Level 2. This brings with it great job satisfaction, but it can also be exhausting at times. For this reason we have acknowledged that taking care of ourselves is just as important as taking care of our clients and their families, as we cannot give endlessly to others if we never receive support in return. Ensure that you have sufficient staff support measures in place and use the team around you wisely.

This chapter is not intended to be 'all you ever need to know'. The hope is that it will offer time to reflect on present practice, celebrate what we do well and inspire you to look further and keep learning more about this fascinating area of nursing care, just as writing this chapter has helped me to look further and learn more. Remember, each of us will, at some point, be the client or the family member. If your care delivery is as good as you would ever hope to receive then that will indeed be the best possible measure of optimal care delivery.

References

Bowlby J. (1969) *Attachment and Loss. Vol. 1 Attachment.* Harmondsworth, Middlesex, Penguin.

Bowlby J. (1973) *Attachment and Loss. Vol. 2 Separation.* Harmondsworth, Middlesex, Penguin.

Brennan J. (2001) Adjustment to cancer – coping or personal transition? *Psycho-oncology,* **10,** 1–18.

Buchan J.E.F. (1995) Nurses' estimations of patients' prognoses in the last days of life. *International Journal of Palliative Nursing,* **1** (1) 12–16.

Burnard P. (1997) *Effective Communication Skills for Health Professionals,* 2nd edn. Cheltenham, Nelson Thornes.

Burnard P. (2005) *Counselling Skills for Health Professionals,* 4th edn. Cheltenham, Nelson Thornes.

Cash T. and Pruzinsky T. (eds) (2002) *Body Image: A Handbook of Theory, Research, and Clinical Practice.* New York, Guilford Press.

Christakis N.A. (1998) Predicting patient survival before and after hospice enrolment. *The Hospice Journal,* **13** (1/2), 78–87.

Cooper T. and Roth I. (eds) (2002) *Challenging Psychological Issues.* Maidenhead, Open University Press/McGraw Hill.

Doyle D. (1999) The provision of palliative care. In: *Oxford Textbook of Palliative Medicine,* 2nd edn (D. Doyle, G.W.C. Hanks and N. MacDonald, eds). Oxford, Oxford University Press, pp. 41–55.

Egan G. (2001) *The Skilled Helper. A Problem-Management and Opportunity-Development Approach to Helping*, 7th edn. Pacific Grove, USA, Brooks/Cole.

Engels G.L. (1980) The clinical application of the biopsychosocial model. *American Journal of Psychiatry*, **137**, 535–544.

Evans C. and McCarthy M. (1985) Prognostic uncertainty in terminal care: Can the Karnofsky Index help? *Lancet*, May 25th, 1204–1206.

FACIT (2005) *The functional assessment of chronic illness therapy (FACIT) measurement system overview.* http://www.facit.org/about/overview_measure.aspx

Freud A. and Dann S. (1951) An experiment in group upbringing. In: *Psychoanalytic Study of the Child*, Vol. 6 (R.S. Eisler and A. Freud, eds). New York, International Universities Press, pp. 127–168.

Field D. and Copp G. (1999) Communication and awareness about the dying in the 1990s. *Palliative Medicine*, **13** (6), 459–468.

Foley K.M. and Gelband H. (eds) (2001) *Improving Palliative Care for Cancer*. Washington DC, National Academies Press.

Glaser B.G. and Strauss A.L. (1965) *Awareness of Dying*. Chicago, Aldine.

Gott C.M., Ahmedzai S.H. and Wood C. (2001) How many patients at an acute hospital have palliative care needs? Comparing the perspectives of medical and nursing staff. *Palliative Medicine*, **15** (6), 451–460.

Gross R.D. (1993) *Psychology. The Science of Mind and Behaviour*, 2nd edn. London. Hodder & Stoughton.

Hargie O. (1991) *Effective Communication Skills for Health Professionals*, 2nd edn. London, Routledge.

Heyse-Moore L.H. and Johnson-Bell V.E. (1987) Can doctors accurately predict the life-expectancy of patients with terminal cancer. *Palliative Medicine*, **1** (3), 165–166.

MacAdam D.B. and Smith M. (1987) An initial assessment of suffering in terminal illness. *Palliative Medicine*, **1** (1), 37–47.

National Institute for Clinical Excellence (2004) *Guidance on Cancer Services: Improving Supportive and Palliative Care for Adults with Cancer*. London, NICE.

Ogden J. (2000) *Health Psychology. A Textbook*. Maidenhead, Open University Press/ McGraw Hill.

Parkes C.M. (1972) Accuracy of predications of survival in later stages of cancer. *British Medical Journal*, **2**, 29–31.

Price B. (1990a) A model for body-image care. *Journal of Advanced Nursing*, **15** (5), 3.

Price B. (1990b) *Body image. Nursing Concepts and Care*. London, Prentice Hall.

Rotter J.B. (1966) Generalised expectancies for internal versus external locus of control of reinforcement. *Psychological Monographs*, **30** (1), 1–26.

Scherer K.R. (1996) Emotion. In: *Introduction to Social Psychology. A European Perspective*, 2nd edn (M. Hewstone, W. Stroebe and G.M. Stephenson, eds). Oxford, Blackwell Publishing.

Schilder P. (1935) *Image and Appearance of the Human Body*. London, Kegan Paul.

Snaith R.P. (2003) The Hospital Anxiety and Depression Scale. *Health and Quality of life Outcomes*, **1**, 29.

Stroebe W. and Jonas K. (1996) Principles of attitude formation and strategies of change. In: *Introduction to Social Psychology. A European Perspective*, 2nd edn (M. Hewstone, W. Stroebe and G.M. Stephenson, eds). Oxford, Blackwell Publishing.

Swindle R., Heller K., Pescosolido B. and Kikuzawa S. (2000) Responses to nervous breakdowns in America over a 40 year period: Mental health policy implications. *American Psychological Association*, **55**, 740–747.

Twycross R. and Lichter I. (1999) The terminal phase. In: *Oxford Textbook of Palliative Medicine*, 2nd edn (D. Doyle, G.W.C. Hanks and N. MacDonald, eds). Oxford, Oxford University Press, pp. 977–995.

Wood C., Littleton K. and Oates J. (2002) Lifespan development. In: *Challenging Psychological Issues* (T. Cooper and I. Roth, eds). Milton Keynes, The Open University.

Woods S. (1998) Holism in nursing. In: *Philosophical Issues in Nursing Practice* (S.D. Edwards, ed.). London, Macmillan Press.

Viganò A., Dorgan M., Bruera E. and Suarez–Almazor M.E. (1999) The relative accuracy of clinical estimation of the duration of life for patients with end of life cancer. *Cancer*, **86** (1), 170–176.

Zabora J.R. (1998) Screening procedures for psychosocial distress. In: *Psycho-oncology* (J.C. Holland, W. Breitbart, P.B. Jacobsen, *et al.*, eds). New York, Oxford University Press, pp. 653–661.

Zigmond A.S. and Snaith R.P. (1983) The Hospital Anxiety and Depression Scale. *Acta Psychiatrica Scandinavica*, **67** (6), 361–370.

Chapter 5
Evaluating Rehabilitation Services

Rebecca Jester

The aim of this chapter is to critically discuss comprehensive evaluation of rehabilitation services. Indicative content within this chapter includes:

- Justification for evaluation
- Setting up and evaluating nurse-led services
- Defining patient outcomes
- Disease-specific and generic health and quality-of-life outcomes
- Psychometric properties of outcome measures
- Patient satisfaction as a legitimate measure of outcome
- Economic evaluation of rehabilitation services

Justification for evaluation

The genesis of clinical governance (DH, 1998) has necessitated the systematic collection of patient outcome data using valid and reliable methods to evaluate health service provision. Prior to clinical governance, the collection of outcome data was somewhat *ad hoc*, with individual clinicians taking unilateral decisions about what data should be collected, if any. Collection of outcome data within rehabilitation is necessary:

- To evaluate the effectiveness of particular treatment modalities
- As an integral part of patient assessment, to inform diagnoses
- To compare alternative treatment interventions
- To provide feedback to patients and their families on progress

As clinicians supporting rehabilitation clients and their families, we need to develop and implement robust and systematic approaches to the evaluation of outcome/s. The approach needs to be multidisciplinary and must include the client themself as an active participant, rather than as a passive recipient of evaluation. The evaluation approach needs to be multidimensional and should include: disease specific and generic quality-of-life measures; patient satisfaction; and economic evaluation.

Setting up and evaluating nurse-led services

Many of those taking on advancing roles, such as nurse consultants and specialist nurse practitioners, develop their own nurse-led services. This may be to replace services currently provided by other members of the multidisciplinary team, for example medics, or to meet an unmet patient need. The development of nurse-led services needs careful planning and organisation. The first stage is to develop a proposal for the service, which needs to address the following issues:

- What is the rationale for the development of the service?
- Is it replacing an existing service or is it a new provision?
- Who will be delivering the service and has the individual/s the necessary experience and education to deliver the service?
- What additional resources are required to set up the service?
- What are the anticipated benefits of the development?
- Are protocols, guidelines or directives required?
- How will the service be evaluated?
- What are the issues around vicarious liability?
- Who will be involved in the planning of the service (user involvement, members of the multidisciplinary team, managers, representatives from primary care trusts, general practitioners, administrators and finance personal)?

This list is not meant to be exhaustive, but simply a guide to the main issues that need to be considered. As with any change, it is important that those who may be affected be kept informed of developments and actively involved in the decision-making process. The development of nurse-led services, particularly those replacing services previously provided by medical staff, may be met with resistance from some clinicians and patients. This should be minimised by involving the stakeholders in the change process and by providing empirical evidence of why the nurse-led service will improve efficiency and quality of health care provision.

Once the proposal for the development has been accepted it is important that patients understand they will be seen by an advanced nurse practitioner (ANP), rather than a doctor. This can be explained in the letter asking them to attend the clinic. When patients access the service the nurse practitioner must reinforce their role to ensure the validity of any consent to carry out a procedure. Also, it is essential that your service is adequately resourced. From my own experience as an ANP, an assistant or nurse was not initially assigned to my clinic, as I was a nurse. This meant having to collect patient notes/X-rays, sorting out transport if a patient needed to be scanned at another site or arranging admission. A consultant medical colleague would not be expected to do these duties as well as assess, diagnose and treat a full complement of patients!

Evaluation of any nurse-led service is essential to establish its effectiveness. In addition, it may be appropriate to compare service provision between nurse-led and medically led interventions in terms of both cost and effectiveness, especially when the new intervention may have been approved on a time-limited pilot basis. The precise details of what should be included in a comprehensive evaluation will vary depending on the nature of the service being provided. However, it is reasonable to expect an evaluation to include the following:

- Ascertaining patient satisfaction
- Measuring patient outcomes
- Auditing the nature and number of complications
- Reviewing the nature and number of complaints
- Determining the cost of the service
- Auditing waiting times and 'do not attends'
- Establishing the views of other members of the multidisciplinary team on the service

Patient satisfaction, patient outcomes and economic evaluation will be discussed in detail within this chapter to provide a theoretical evidence-based approach to evaluating nurse-led interventions.

Defining patient outcomes

Historically, outcome measures can be traced back to Florence Nightingale, who devised a system for comparing death rates by diagnostic category during the Crimean war (Pynsent *et al.*, 1993). Bulstrode (1993) described outcomes as being a measure of change, the endpoint being compared with the situation prior to an intervention such as therapy or surgery; and having relative value rather than being an absolute. Several methods are available for measuring patient outcomes, including (Bowling, 2001):

- Physical tests of function
- Direct observation of behaviour
- Patient interview

There are advantages and disadvantages to the above methods of measuring outcome. For example, physical tests of function conducted by a clinician – such as assessing passive and active range of joint movement, muscle strength and deep tendon reflexes – are objective measures. However, they are susceptible to poor inter-rater reliability and do not capture the impact of the disease on the patient. Direct observation of behaviour may be intrusive to patients, and may only provide a 'snapshot' of patient ability unless carried out regularly and at different times of the day/night. Patient interview typically involves asking patients their views on their condition and to complete self-report measures of functional ability. For a proportion of rehabilitation patients this may not be possible due to difficulties with communication or cognition.

Self-report measures contain an inherent component of subjectivity. However, this should not be viewed as a limitation, as the subjectivity provides the strength of this type of measure, which aims to capture the individual's perception of their own health. Individuals 'may react differently to apparently similar levels of physical impairment, depending on their expectations, priorities and prior experience' (Bowling, 1997; p. 17). Also, it is has been reported that there may be discrepancy between clinicians' and patients' perceptions of health status, with many clinicians overestimating the impact of a particular treatment or intervention. However, it has been suggested that patient self-report measures of function/health have their limitations. Pynsent *et al.* (1993) suggested, 'Patients' memories can be poor and when comparing their condition prior to a procedure/treatment to that afterwards the patient may genuinely have difficulty in remembering what their condition was like prior to the intervention' (p. 8).

Disease-specific and generic health and quality-of-life outcomes

Self-report measures of health and disease can be subclassified into two main groups: disease-specific, and generic quality-of-life measures. Generic measures of health aim to measure the multifaceted nature of health and well being, so they should be comprehensive and include items relating to social and psychological health as well as physical health (Bowling, 2005). Also, generic measures enable comparison of the impact of an intervention across different patient groups.

Generic measures aim to evaluate a client's general quality of life, but what is quality of life? Certainly self-evaluation of how good one's life is will be influenced by many factors, including their cultural, religious and social background. In western society there is an increasing emphasis on longevity and material wealth. However, as clinicians we must be sensitive to the fact that each individual client will have their own unique perceptions of what constitutes quality of life for them. One of the major constraints of generic measures is that they lack specificity and sensitivity, and are unable to identify the condition-specific aspects of a disease that are essential for measuring outcomes.

It is for these reasons many experts recommend that generic measures be supplemented with condition-specific measures. Examples of disease-specific and generic quality-of-life measures are provided in Tables 5.1 and 5.2 and also within the condition-specific chapters.

Table 5.1 Examples of disease-specific measures.

Name of tool	Specific disease or body system	Authors	Description
Western Ontario and McMaster Universities Arthritis Index (WOMAC)	Osteoarthritis	Bellamy *et al.* (1988)	The visual analogue version is quite difficult for older patients to comprehend. So the Likert scale version is preferable. The tool has been subjected to rigorous validation studies.
Barthel Index	Neuromuscular or musculoskeletal disorders, but tends to be used generally for patients undergoing rehabilitation	Mahoney and Barthel (1965)	The original index lacked sensitivity and specificity, but modified versions by either Shah *et al.* (1989) or Granger's Modified Index (1984) have much improved psychometric properties.
Beck Depression Inventory (BDI)	Depression	Beck *et al.* (1961)	Can be used as a self-report measure or administered by a clinician. Relatively short (21 items) and easy to analyse results.
Guyatt's Chronic Heart-failure Questionnaire (CHQ)	Heart failure/ shortness of breath	Guyatt *et al.* (1988)	Comprises 19 questions with Likert scale responses, e.g. all of the time to none of the time, covers dyspnoea during activities, fatigue and emotional function.
St George's Respiratory Questionnaire (SGRQ)	Chronic obstructive airways disease (COAD) and asthma	Quirk and Jones (1990)	Well-validated tool comprising 76 items. It does not include items around anxiety and depression, which are relatively common in this client group.

Table 5.1 does not assume to constitute an in-depth analysis of all disease-specific measures used either in the UK or internationally, but rather to give you a taste of the types of assessment tools available.

Psychometric properties of outcome measures

When deciding upon a particular tool to assess patient outcome it is imperative that the evidence-base underpinning the development and validation of the tool is analysed. You need to consider the validity, reliability, specificity, sensitivity and practicability of the tool. A definition of each of these terms is provided below:

Table 5.2 Examples of generic health and quality-of-life outcome measures.

Name of tool	Author	Description
Short Form – 36 Health Survey Questionnaire (SF 36)	Ware (1993)	Relatively brief and comprehensive tool. Comprises 36 items and can be interviewer-administered face-to-face or by telephone, or completed by the patient on their own. Has well proven validity and reliability.
Nottingham Health Profile	Hunt (1984)	One of the most commonly used measures of broader health status. Psychometric properties well established, particularly for patients suffering with severe chronic conditions such as heart failure.
Sickness Impact Profile (SIP)	Gilson *et al.* (1979)	Comprises 2 overall domains (physical and psychosocial) with 12 categories and a total of 136 items. Can be used as a self-report measure or by interviewer administration and takes approximately 20–30 minutes to complete.
Dartmouth COOP Function Charts	Nelson *et al.* (1993)	Brief functional health assessment charts, which are short and easy to administer.
Rosser Index of Disability	Rosser (1992)	Originally developed as a basic tool to calculate quality-of-life years. Health index where patients are graded into 1 of 8 areas of disability (none to unconscious or negative scores for PVS)

- **Validity**: the degree to which a test measures what it is intended to measure. There are four types of validity: construct, content, face and predictive.
- **Reliability**: the degree to which a test measures the same attribute each time it is used. We also need to consider inter-rater reliability, which refers to the degree to which two or more assessors agree in their use of the measurement tool. For example, if two practitioners complete the modified Barthel Index with the same patient within 10 minutes of each other we would expect the score to be the same or very similar, equating to a high degree of inter-rater reliability.
- **Specificity**: defined as the proportion of all negative cases that are correctly identified as negative, i.e. the test will be negative in patients who do not have the attribute (the false-positive rate).
- **Sensitivity**: the ability of a measuring tool to make fine discriminations between objects with differing amounts of the attribute being measured. For example, the original Barthel Index lacked sensitivity because for most activities of daily living categories one could only assign either 'totally independent' or 'totally dependent'.
- **Practicability**: how user-friendly the tool is in terms of administration and scoring.

Copyright restrictions on instruments vary. Some measures can be used freely, whilst others require the author's permission. Many authors permit clinicians to administer the tool without a charge, but others can only be obtained by paying a fee. It is wise to contact the original author to check on copyright restriction prior to using the tool in practice or for research purposes. Also remember that if you amend a tool you will need to conduct a pilot study to re-affirm its psychometric properties.

It is important to consider by whom, when and how disease-specific and generic health and quality-of-life measures should be administered. They form a useful adjunct to initial history taking and clinical examination, and will provide a baseline to measure against during the patient's rehabilitative journey. The multidisciplinary team in liaison with the patient must include regular re-administration of the tool/s at agreed evaluation points in the patient's rehabilitation plan. It is important to seek guidance on the frequency of administration of the tool from the validation literature, and to ensure all team members have been properly educated on the administration and analysis of results.

Patient satisfaction as a legitimate measure of outcome

Providers of health care are now increasingly expected to supply information regarding patient outcomes and to demonstrate clinical effectiveness (DH, 1998) following various treatment interventions. In addition to quantitative health outcome measures, such as mortality, morbidity, incidence of complications and re-admission rates, as well as length of stay and functional improvements, patient satisfaction is considered to be a valid outcome measure (Walsh & Walsh, 1999). This was affirmed by Greenfield *et al.* (1985) who stated, 'patients' views should be viewed as a legitimate, important measure of quality of care and an indirect measure of health outcome' (cited in Hardy *et al.*, 1996; p. 65).

However, patient satisfaction is more than merely a customer relations exercise. Patients' participation in their care, and satisfaction with care-delivery directly impact on treatment compliance and their well being (Ley, 1990; Bowling, 2005). Ley (1990) suggested there are two main reasons why patient satisfaction is important. Firstly, 'that patient satisfaction is a goal in its own right and secondly that patient satisfaction is an important determinant of patients' compliance with advice' (p. 1). Hardy *et al.* (1996) expanded upon these assertions, suggesting there are three important reasons for ascertaining patient satisfaction:

- Patient satisfaction is known to be associated with a better health outcome
- Dissatisfied patients are often unable to take their custom elsewhere
- The development of a consumer-based service model of health care

Bowling (1992) suggested that, 'satisfaction can affect compliance with, and acceptance of treatment and outcome of care' (p. 32). Dissatisfied patients may not comply with treatment regimes due to poor communication between patient and health care professional. Poor or non-compliance with treatment can have a severe negative impact on patient progress and recovery. Ley (1990) focused on the triad of communication, satisfaction and compliance with regards to their impact upon each other; suggesting that poor communication between patients and health care practitioners results in patient dissatisfaction, which, in turn, results in poor or non-compliance with medical advice and treatment.

Fitzpatrick & Hopkins (1993) stated that, 'a number of studies have found that satisfied patients are more likely to follow the advice they receive or adhere to treatment regimes' (p. 4). Hall *et al.* (1990) discussed the positive impact of satisfaction on health, and suggested there are two possible reasons for this. Firstly, 'that satisfied patients are more likely to adhere to medical advice and secondly that satisfaction has a placebo type effect on psychological well being, which in turn has a positive effect on physical health' (p. 24). Therefore, it may be deduced that dissatisfied patients will experience stress and anxiety with a subsequent negative impact on their physical well being. The negative impact of psychological distress on health is well documented, specifically relating to effects on the immune and cardiovascular systems (Atkinson *et al.*, 1990). Despite the wealth of evidence to support the importance of patient satisfaction there is some scepticism regarding the validity of patient satisfaction as a measure of outcome. Walsh & Walsh (1999) suggested that, 'satisfaction has such an elusive and subjective quality that it means different things to different people' (p. 308). In addition, some personality types may never be satisfied. Therefore, careful deliberation of what constitutes satisfaction with health care is imperative.

It is important that patient satisfaction is viewed as a valuable measure of quality of care and that valid and reliable psychometric measures are used. It is for this reason that patient satisfaction should be an important aspect of evaluating and comparing nurse-led services in rehabilitation. In reality, patients cannot generally vote with their feet as the NHS has a monopoly over health care provision, except for the few who can afford private health care. Therefore it is essential to ensure that any intervention is evaluated in terms of patient satisfaction in addition to professionals' views of outcome.

Defining patient satisfaction

Patient satisfaction was described by Pascoe (1983) as, 'patients' reactions to salient aspects of the context, process and results of their experience' (p. 185). Some researchers (e.g. Wolf *et al.* (1978) and Walsh & Walsh (1999)) have chosen to focus on satisfaction with a particular health care professional, such as the physician or nurse, instead of overall satisfaction with the whole experience of health care. Wolf *et al.* (1978) examined three aspects of satisfaction with physician intervention using their Medical Interview Satisfaction Scale, i.e.:

- The cognitive aspect – essentially the quality and amount of information provided by the doctor.

- The affective aspect – the amount that the patient feels that the doctor listens, understands and is interested in them.
- The behavioural aspect – the patient's evaluation of the doctor's competence.

Walsh & Walsh (1999) described the use of the Newcastle Satisfaction with Nursing Scale (NSNS), which examines patients' satisfaction with a variety of dimensions of nursing activity and attitude, such as nurses' empathy toward patients and level of competence. However, the development and theoretical base of the NSNS is given scant attention in terms of psychometric validity.

Patient satisfaction with nursing as an accurate predictor of overall satisfaction with the quality of treatment and care is affirmed by a recent Canadian study measuring patient satisfaction across 14 hospitals in Ontario (Laschinger *et al.*, 2005). However, the value of ascertaining satisfaction with just one professional group is limited. A patient may report being highly satisfied with their interactions with one particular professional group but feel generally dissatisfied with their total health care experience.

Ley (1990) stated that investigators had concentrated on specific aspects of patient satisfaction. For example, some investigators had focused on satisfaction with various aspects of communication between patient and health care professionals, e.g. information giving practices by health care professionals as a strong predictor of patient satisfaction. Again this may be viewed as a reductionist model of evaluating patient satisfaction by focusing on a single indicator, i.e. communication rather than taking a holistic approach examining satisfaction with the total care experience. Fitzpatrick & Hopkins (1993) suggested that patient satisfaction had, 'proved to be a multidimensional construct' (p. 36). Hall & Dornan (1988) delineated eleven aspects of patient satisfaction, which are presented in Table 5.3. These were derived from a series of open-ended interviews with a sample of adult inpatients and subsequent content analysis. Furthermore, the complex and multifaceted nature of patient satisfaction in contemporary health care has been confirmed by Bowling (2005).

The early work of Wolf *et al.* (1978) and Hall & Dornan (1988) suggested that there are underpinning psychological components within 'satisfaction' such as those mentioned in Table 5.3. This was corroborated by Hardy *et al.* (1996) who stressed the importance of having a theoretical orientation to the measures

Table 5.3 Components of patient satisfaction (Hall and Dornan, 1988).

• Humaneness	• Access
• Informativeness	• Cost
• Overall quality	• Facilities
• Competence	• Health outcome
• Attention to psychosocial problems	• Continuity
• Bureaucracy	

of patient satisfaction, which should be based upon data derived from sound factor analysis of psychometric data about patient satisfaction. Rubin (1990) identified three domains of patient satisfaction:

- Health improvement
- Affective state (e.g. anxiety and depression)
- Sense of safety and security

Hardy & West (1994) elaborated on the work of Rubin (1990), developing a patient satisfaction measure embracing theories of organisational participation and socialisation called the 'Hospital Patient Satisfaction Index' (HPSI). The HPSI underwent rigorous piloting within two large NHS hospitals with a total sample of 713 patients who were representative of a wide range of adult specialties.

Forbes & Brown (1995) proposed that patients' perceptions of satisfaction 'will vary depending on gender, age, social status, education level, cultural background and previous experiences with health care' (p. 737). Hence, testing of tools must encompass a sufficient sample to cover this range of patient characteristics. Bowling (1992) critically discussed the influence of social class on satisfaction, stating: 'Satisfaction is generally concentrated in social classes 1 and 5, reflecting the greater ability of those in social class one to choose their care, and the greater acceptance of low standards among the lower social classes' (p. 32). The age of patients in relation to level of satisfaction was given particular mention by Bowling (1992), stating: 'older people are generally stated to be less critical of their care'. It is evident from the literature that patient satisfaction is a multidimensional concept, which includes physical, social and psychological components (Rubin, 1990; Hall & Dornan, 1983). In addition, it would appear that focusing on only one particular aspect of patient satisfaction – such as satisfaction with one professional group, e.g. nurses or doctors – or focusing on communication practices would appear to adopt a reductionist approach to ascertaining patient satisfaction. Therefore it is important that measurement of patient satisfaction should be multidimensional and endorse the biographical differences such as gender and age.

Effective measurement of patient satisfaction

Many tools designed to measure patient satisfaction lack validity and reliability. The factors that may predict patient satisfaction are difficult to identify due to the subjective nature of satisfaction. In addition, patient satisfaction ratings 'consistently achieve high scores, due to a lack of sensitivity and inability to accurately identify components of satisfaction' (Walsh & Walsh, 1999; p. 308). Predominantly, measures of patient satisfaction have been managerially developed and administered within the NHS (Fitzpatrick & Hopkins, 1993). Consequently, these measures have focused on physical amenities, hotel aspects of care and process indicators such as waiting times, which are within the remit of NHS management. This type of satisfaction measure, however, fails to address the fundamental psychological components of satisfaction and process and outcome of clinical aspects of care as discussed earlier. This was affirmed by Forbes and Brown (1995), 'Satisfaction surveys mainly focus on criteria established by institutions that may not reflect what is important to patients' (p. 737).

McDaniel and Nash (1990) examined 21 measures of patient satisfaction with nursing care (PSNC) and, 'found only 9 had psychometrics which had been established with formal procedures' (p. 183). This supports the importance of establishing the development procedures and academic underpinning of satisfaction measures prior to their administration and analysis to ensure validity and reliability. Additionally, the practicability of satisfaction measures must be given careful attention. Questionnaires should not be too onerous for patients to complete, which may lead to unsatisfactory completion and ethical compromise of data collection.

When to measure patient satisfaction

Ley (1975) reported 'a curvi-linear relationship between the percentage of patients reporting satisfaction and the time elapsing since discharge from hospital or following a consultation' (p. 9). Ley (1975) purported that levels of satisfaction are higher within one week of discharge from hospital than measures taken between two and four weeks after discharge, but that levels of satisfaction rise at eight weeks following discharge. This refutes the earlier work by Spelman *et al.* (1966) who reported that satisfaction increased with increasing time since discharge. It should be considered that hospitalised patients are generally experiencing stress due to a culmination of ill health and being separated from family, home and their own routine. This may influence the correlation between timing and rates of satisfaction as patients' stress diminishes on return to their home.

In addition, it is imperative that those who collect patient satisfaction data remain neutral, and that patients participating in patient satisfaction research are assured of confidentiality and anonymity. This was affirmed by Fitzpatrick & Hopkins (1993): 'Neutrality of data gatherers must be guaranteed and confidentiality assured' (p. 8). To ensure the neutrality of data collection, the advanced nurse practitioners must ensure that an independent individual administers and collects data pertaining to patient satisfaction with their service.

Economic evaluation

No government or authority is likely to favour health innovations that will probably be more costly than existing health care provisions. Investigating cost-effectiveness is an essential component of a comprehensive evaluation of the suitability and acceptability of nurse-led interventions.

It is important to define the term 'cost-effective' prior to embarking upon a review of methods of economic analysis of health care interventions. Doubilet *et al.* (1986) have provided a comprehensive definition of the term 'cost-effective', suggesting it should be used for cases in which: 'one strategy is more cost-effective than another if it is (a) less costly and at least as effective; (b) more effective and more costly, its additional benefit being worth its additional cost; or (c) less effective and less costly, the added benefit of the rival strategy not being worth its extra cost' (p. 254).

Donaldson *et al.* (1996) suggested that economic evaluation techniques cannot be predetermined until the results of a parallel investigation into the effectiveness of the intervention are known.

Several methods can be used to evaluate the cost-effectiveness of health care interventions, these include: cost-minimisation analysis (CMA); cost–benefit analysis (CBA) and cost-effectiveness analysis (CEA).

Cost-minimisation analysis

Cost-minimisation analysis calculates the difference in monetary terms between two interventions (e.g. nurse- versus medically led services) assuming that both interventions are equally effective in terms of outcome. Therefore, the intervention that costs less is considered to be more cost-effective (Gold *et al.*, 1996).

Cost–benefit analysis

'In CBA both the benefits and the costs of an intervention are measured in monetary terms, the CBA then offers a bottom-line of a benefit–cost ratio in monetary figures' (Beauchamp & Childress, 2001). Monetary value is apportioned to health consequences by calculating willingness to pay and human capital. Willingness to pay is assessed via surveying opinions relating to trade-offs between health and money. Human capital is calculated on the basis of the 'produce value of people in the economy' (Gold *et al.*, 1996). CBA involves apportioning a monetary figure, in the UK in pounds sterling, to improvements in outcome. For example, calculating the monetary value of how reduced joint stiffness would equate to a reduced consumption of analgesic and anti-inflammatory medication (monetary value) or how patients would claim less mobility allowance, etc. However, CBA can be used as a framework to identify the trade-offs between cost and benefit without converting benefit into monetary terms (Donaldson *et al.*, 1996). Donaldson *et al.* (1996) suggested the 'CBA framework can be used to lay out the information on costs and benefits to aid a decision about whether any gains provided by the experimental treatment are worth the extra costs involved. This may be as far as the economic evaluation can take it' (p. 268). The CBA model appears to endorse ethical principles of balancing benefits, such as improvement in health, against monetary cost.

Cost-effectiveness analysis

The purpose of CEA is to compare the relative value of two or more interventions in achieving better health or outcomes. 'The results of such evaluations are typically summarised in a cost-effectiveness ratio, where the denominator reflects the gain in health achieved and the numerator reflects the cost of obtaining that health gain' (Gold *et al.*, 1996; p. 18). However, when one of the interventions under study is both more effective and less costly than the alternative, there is no need to calculate a cost-effectiveness ratio.

CEA is described as a tool for improving social welfare by maximising the aggregate health effect achievable at the lowest possible cost (Gold *et al.*, 1996). The theoretical foundations of CEA encompass welfare economics, which endorses the sociological principles of utilitarianism. Cost-effective analysis provides a method of comparing interventions so that decision-makers can maximise health benefits with finite resources. Furthermore, CEA proposes that any alteration in the mode of health care delivery produces both economic and social consequences, i.e. development of nurse-led services.

What should be included within an economic evaluation of nurse-led services?

Calculating and comparing costs for nurse-led services is complex. It must encompass cost incurred by patients and families as well as any shift in cost from tertiary to community and outpatient services.

Literature relating to economic analysis suggests that several types of data should be collected when estimating cost in a CEA, which include both direct and indirect costs (Donaldson *et al.*, 1996). Direct costs apply to items such as clinical investigations, medications, nursing and therapy interventions and patient, transport, e.g. ambulance journeys. Indirect costs relate to items such as the overhead costs of running a hospital or clinic: for example, utility costs, maintenance of the building and administration. However, it is important not just to examine the direct and indirect costs related to the tertiary centre, but in addition to monitor whether there is a shift in costs to community and outpatient services. For example, if following consultation at a nurse-led orthopaedic clinic the patient has to visit their general practitioner to obtain a prescription for a change of analgesia this increases the cost for primary care compared to a medically led clinic, where the prescription would be issued and dispensed by the hospital. This emphasises the importance of nurse practitioners being able to have relevant prescribing authority.

The complexity of ensuring that all relevant costs are included within an economic evaluation necessitates the use of a structured framework underpinned by theoretical relevance, rather than an *ad hoc* approach.

Conclusions

This chapter has discussed the importance of robust and comprehensive evaluation of rehabilitation services, with a specific emphasis on the setting up and evaluation of services led by advanced nurses. An overview of disease-specific and generic quality-of-life measures has been presented and I would suggest the following as further reading on this topic: Bowling (2001, 2005).

It may be a useful exercise to review the evaluation tools currently used within your rehabilitation team and to ascertain their psychometric properties.

References

Atkinson R., Atkinson R., Smith E., Bem D. and Hilgard E. (1990) *Introduction to Psychology*, 10th edn. London, Harcourt Brace Jovanovich Publishing.

Beauchamp T. and Childress J. (2001) *Principles of Biomedical Ethics*, 5th edn. Oxford, Oxford University Press.

Beck A., Ward C. and Mendelson M. (1961) An inventory for measuring depression. *Archives of General Psychiatry*, **4**, 561–71.

Bellamy N., Buchanan W., Goldsmith C., Campbell J. and Stitt L. (1988) Validation study of WOMAC: a health status instrument for measuring clinically important patient-relevant outcomes following total hip or knee arthroplasty in osteoarthritis. *Journal of Orthopaedics and Rheumatology*, **1**, 95–108.

Bowling A. (1992) Assessing health needs and measuring patient satisfaction. *Nursing Time*, **88**, 31.

Bowling A. (1997) *Measuring Health. A Review of Quality of Life Measurement Scales*, 2nd edn. Maidenhead, Open University Press.

Bowling A. (2001) *Measuring Disease*, 2nd edn. Maidenhead, Open University Press.

Bowling A. (2005) *Measuring Health: A Review of Quality of Life Measurement Scales*, 3rd edn. Maidenhead, Open University Press.

Bulstrode C. (1993) Outcome measures and their analysis. In: *Outcome Measures in Orthopaedics* (P. Pynsent, J. Fairbank and A. Carr, eds). Oxford, Butterworth–Heinemann.

Department of Health (1998) *The New NHS. Modern and Dependable: A National Framework for Assessing Performance*. London, NHSE.

Donaldson C., Hundley V. and McIntosh E. (1996) Using economics alongside clinical trials: why we cannot choose the evaluation technique in advance. *Health Economics*, **5**, 267–269.

Doubilet P., Weinstein M.C. and McNeil B.J. (1986) Use and misuse of the term 'cost effective' in medicine. *New England Journal of Medicine*, **314**, 253–256.

Fitzpatrick R. and Hopkins A. (1993) *Measurement of Patients' Satisfaction with their Care*. London, Royal College of Physicians.

Forbes M. and Brown J. (1995) Developing an instrument for measuring patient satisfaction. *Association of Operating Room Nurses Journal*, **61** (4), 737–743.

Gilson B., Bergner M. and Bobbitt R. (1979) *The Sickness Impact Profile: Final Development and Testing*. Washington, University of Washington Press.

Gold M., Siegel J., Russell L. and Weinstein M. (1996) *Cost-Effectiveness in Health and Medicine*. Oxford, Oxford University Press.

Granger C. and McNamara M. (1984) Functional assessment utilisation: The Long Range Evaluation System. In: *Functional Assessment in Rehabilitation Medicine* (C. Granger and G. Gresham, eds). Baltimore, MD, Williams & Williams.

Greenfield S., Kaplan S. and Ware J. (1985) Expanding patient involvement in care. *Annals of Internal Medicine*, **102**, 520–528.

Guyatt G., Sullivan M. and Fallen E. (1988) A controlled trial of digoxin in heart failure. *American Journal of Cardiology*, **61**, 371–375.

Hall J. and Dornan M. (1988) What patients think about their medical care and how often they are asked: a meta-analysis of the satisfaction literature. *Social Science and Medicine*, **27**, 935–939.

Hall J., Feldstein M. and Fretwell M. (1990) Older patients health status and satisfaction with medical care in an HMO population. *Medical Care*, **28**, 261–270.

Hardy G. and West M. (1994) Patient satisfaction. Happy talk. *Health Service Journal*, **104**, 24–26.

Hardy G.E., West M.A. and Hill F. (1996) Components and predictors of patient satisfaction. *British Journal of Health Psychology*, **1**, 65–85.

Hunt S. (1984) Nottingham Health Profile. In: *Assessment of Quality of Life in Clinical Trials of Cardiovascular Therapies* (M. Wenger, C. Mattson, C. Furberg and J. Elinson, eds). New York, Le Jacq.

Laschinger H., Hall L., Pedersen C. and Almost J. (2005) A psychometric analysis of the patient satisfaction with nursing care quality: an actionable approach to measuring patient satisfaction. *Journal of Nursing Care Quality*, **20** (3), 220–230.

Ley P. (1975) Complaints by hospital staff and patients: a review of the literature. *Bulletin of the British Psychology Society*, **25**, 115–120.

Ley P. (1990) *Communicating with Patients: Improving Communication, Satisfaction and Compliance*. London, Chapman and Hall.

Mahoney F. and Barthel D. (1965) Functional evaluation: The Barthel Index. *Maryland State Medical Journal*, **14**, 61–65.

McDaniel C. and Nash J. (1990) Compendium of instruments. Measuring patient satisfaction with nursing care. *Quarterly Review Bulletin*, **May**, 182–188.

Nelson E., Landgraf J. and Hays D. (1993) The COOP Function Charts: A system to measure patient function in physicians' offices. [Cited in: Bowling A., ed. (1995) *Measuring Disease*. Maidenhead, Open University Press.]

Pascoe G. (1983) Patient satisfaction in primary health care. A literature review and analysis. *Evaluation and Program Planning*, **6**, 185–210.

Pynsent P., Fairbank J. and Carr A. (1993) *Outcome Measures in Orthopaedics*. Oxford, Butterworth–Heinemann.

Quirk F. and Jones P. (1990) Patients' perceptions of distress due to symptoms and effects of asthma on daily living and an investigation of possible influential factors. *Clinical Science*, **79**, 17–21.

Rosser R. (1992) Index of health-related quality of life. In: *Measures of the Quality of Life and the Uses to which Such Measures may be Put* (A. Hopkins, ed.). London, Royal College of Physicians.

Rubin J. (1990) Patient evaluation of hospital care: A review of the literature. *Medical Care Supplement*, **28**, 3–9.

Shah S., Vanclay F. and Cooper B. (1989) Improving the sensitivity of the Barthel Index for stroke rehabilitation. *Journal of Clinical Epidemiology*, **42**, 703–709.

Spelman M., Ley P. and Jones C. (1966) How do we improve doctor–patient communications in our hospitals? *World Hospitals*, **2**, 126–134.

Walsh M. and Walsh A. (1999) Measuring patient satisfaction with nursing care: experience of using the Newcastle Satisfaction with Nursing Scale. *Journal of Advanced Nursing*, **29** (2), 307–315.

Ware J. (1993) Measuring patients' views: the optimum measure. *British Medical Journal*, **306**, 1429–1430.

Wolf M., Putnam S., James S. and Stiles W. (1978) The Medical Interview Satisfaction Scale: Development of a scale to measure patient perception of physician behaviour. *Journal of Behavioural Medicine*, **1**, 391–401.

Further reading

Abramowitz A., Cote A. and Berry E. (1987) Analysing patient satisfaction. A multi-analytical approach. *Quality Review Bulletin*, **13** (4), 122–130.

Doering E. (1983) Factors influencing inpatient satisfaction with care. *Quality Review Bulletin*, **9** (10), 291–299.

McDaniel C. and Nash J. (1990) Compendium of instruments. Measuring patient satisfaction with nursing care. *Quality Review Bulletin*, May, 182–188.

Chapter 6
Preparing and Supporting Informal Carers

Rebecca Jester

Introduction

The aim of this chapter is to critically discuss the role of informal carers in the rehabilitation process and how specialist nurses can prepare and support them. Indicative content within this chapter includes:

- Demographics of informal carers providing support for an elderly, sick or disabled relative.
- An overview of UK legislation regarding health and social services' responsibilities to informal carers.
- Positive and negative aspects of informal caring (psychological, social, economic and physical aspects).
- Identifying carer strain.
- The role of specialist nurses in coordinating and leading the support and preparation of informal carers (including approaches to learning and teaching, providing psychological support, liaison with social services and peripatetic and respite services).

Demographics of informal carers

Defining informal caring

The General House Survey (GHS) defines an informal carer as: 'A person looking after or providing some form of regular service for a sick, handicapped or elderly person living in their own or another household' (Rowlands & Parker, 1998). The Carers (Recognition and Services) Act 1995 (DH, 1995) provides a more prescriptive definition: 'Anyone who is either providing or intending to provide substantial amounts of care on a regular basis for people in receipt of, or who appear to a local authority to require, community care services.' However, what is meant by providing service or care? The most obvious care tasks include help with personal hygiene, dressing and preparing meals, but often informal caring involves hidden support and commitment; including worrying as a care responsibility.

This concept is described well in an Australian qualitative study by Cheung & Hocking (2004). The study explores the complex emotional relationship of responsibility undertaken by spousal carers of patients with multiple sclerosis (MS). Carers reported worrying about: their partner's deteriorating condition; their relationship with their partner; their own health; institutional care; and lack of government support. The difficulty with most definitions of informal caring is that they focus on the physical aspects of care and fail to include emotional commitment. Perhaps a more flexible definition is that offered by Ayling (1993), suggesting that an informal carer is: 'any person looking after another, resulting in the carer losing personal freedom'. As specialist nurses we need to acknowledge the holistic nature of informal caring so that we can offer appropriate education and support to family carers.

The prevalence of informal caring in the UK

As discussed in Chapter 3, following the implementation of the Community Care Act (DH, 1989) there has been a systematic shift away from hospital-based care for rehabilitation patients. This is exemplified through changes in service provision, such as hospital at home schemes, and case management of patients with chronic diseases. Consequently, the amount of care provided by family and friends will continue to rise. According to the 2001 General Population Census there were 5.2 million carers in England and Wales, with 68% of them providing care for up to 19 hours a week. This figure is increased to an estimated 6.8 million informal carers in the UK (Banks, 1999), which affirms the GHS figure that 13% of the population provide a minimum of 5 hours or more of informal care per week. Ayling (1993) estimated that carers 'save the country £25 billion per year', while, according to the carers' information website in May 2006, 'informal carers are unpaid and save the UK £57 billion per year' (www. carersinformation.org.uk). Rowlands & Parker (1998) affirmed the notion of savings to the national budget by stating: 'It is clear that the state could never afford to fund the care provided by family and friends, particularly where 1.7 million people are devoting at least 20 hours per week to caring' (p. 13). Those taking on the role of informal carer range from young children to the very elderly.

Identifying carers is a fundamental precondition to providing them with support. However, accurate identification of carers at an early stage in their caregiving career is problematic, as identified in a Scottish study by Jarvis & Worth (2005). Many informal carers do not receive recognition for their role as they do not meet the criteria set by the Department of Health. In addition, many of the research studies to date exploring the contribution of informal carers draw their samples from populations identified by statutory services. This is problematic as nearly 60% of carers receive no support from these statutory services. Therefore, the first role we have as specialists in rehabilitation is to develop systematic sensitive approaches to identifying informal carers. The study by Jarvis & Worth (2005) included the development of a screening tool to identify carers in a Scottish general practice. The methodology used is extremely useful as it asks open-ended questions and permits a broad definition of informal caring, including the emotional commitment of 'caring about' as well as 'caring for'.

An overview of UK legislation regarding health and social services' responsibilities to informal carers

The debate of whose responsibility it is to provide care for the sick, disabled and elderly is complex, with many societal, economic, political, ethical and cultural considerations. Recognition of the role of informal carers began in the 1980s when Griffiths (1988) stated that: 'families, friends and neighbours are the primary means by which people are enabled to live normal lives in the community setting'. A report by the first carers' impact programme (Powell & Kocher, 1996) highlighted the disparity between service provision to support informal carers. It was evident that support was provided on geographical location and luck rather than on a need basis. The need to support informal carers has culminated in The Carers and Disabled Children's Act, which was introduced in Parliament in January 2000 (DH, 2000). The Act sets out to provide a clear strategy for health and social services to provide collaborative support to informal carers on a need basis. The Act stipulates that informal carers are to be viewed as part of everyone's responsibility within health and social care, rather than relying on discrete specialist initiatives and projects (Banks, 1999). Individual carers' needs are to be assessed at the point of referral and an appropriate support plan implemented and evaluated. The Carers and Disabled Children's Act 2000 involved a new right for carers to an assessment of their own needs and circumstances. Local councils are charged with mandatory duties to carers, including: provision of respite to cover short breaks; direct payments for carers' services; and provision of services directly to carers.

The second Act, The Carers (Equal Opportunities) Act 2004 (DH, 2004) came into force on 1 April 2005. This places further legal obligations on local councils to support carers, including:

- A duty to inform informal carers of their right to an assessment of their needs.
- When assessment of a carer's needs is undertaken, councils must take into account whether the carer works or wishes to work and/or undertakes or wishes to undertake education, training or leisure activities.
- Facilitation of cooperation between authorities in relation to the provision of services required by carers.

However, many informal carers still report a lack of access to respite and support services, inadequate preparation for the caring role and inequity of financial support (Smith *et al.*, 2004). Also, the commitment to supporting carers does not appear to be affirmed in the General Medical Services contract, when only three points from a total of 1050 are allocated to the quality of services provided to support carers. As specialist practitioners we have an important role to play in providing education and training for informal carers, and in liaising with our social work colleagues to ensure early and equitable access to support and financial services.

Positive and negative aspects of informal caring (psychological, social, economic and physical aspects)

The effects of informal caring can be classified under three headings: physical, psychosocial and economic. Table 6.1 summarises the potential negative impact on informal carers under these three headings.

The discussion so far has focused on the potential negative consequences of being an informal carer. Research describing any positive consequences of caregiving is virtually absent in the UK literature. The concept of the extended family has diminished in the UK compared to, for example, Eastern cultures where caring for family members is generally still the norm. However, data from studies of long-term carers in the USA conducted in the 1970s and 1980s reveal a number of positive benefits of caregiving: about 75% of caregivers reporting that their role made them feel useful (Doty, 1986). Two other positive consequences of caregiving noted in research studies are: personal affirmation of the caregiver through the caregiving experience; and personal meaning

Table 6.1 Negative impact of informal caring.

Domain	Potential effects
Physical (physical strain)	• Disturbed sleep/fatigue • Physical strain due to manual handling tasks
Psychosocial (emotional and family strain)	• Stress and anxiety • Social isolation • Adjustments to lifestyle • Family adjustments • Disruption to personal plans • Frustration • Work adjustments
Economic (financial strain)	• Losing income either due to relinquishing overtime, reduction of hours or cessation of employment • Cost of special equipment or adaptations to the home

Table 6.2 Positive aspects of informal caring reported by carers of hospital at home (HaH) patients.

- I felt my relative was more comfortable, relaxed and enjoyed being at home.
- I felt my relative had better and more individualised care than if they had remained in hospital.
- The convenience of not travelling to and from the hospital.
- My relative coming home early enabled others to have their surgery quicker.
- I felt my relative recuperated better and quicker at home than in the hospital.
- The scheme provided a high standard of care.
- Staff were caring, helpful and friendly.
- I enjoyed my relative coming home early.
- I felt more involved and in control of my relative's care.
- High frequency of visits by HaH team.
- I felt able to contact the HaH team easily.
- I felt relaxed enough to leave my relative alone for short periods.
- I felt well informed by the HaH team and received good information from them.

through caring for a family member (Lawton, 1989). Montenko (1989), in a study of wives caring for their husbands with Alzheimer's disease, found that continuity and maintaining a sense of sustaining the marital relationship were important positive consequences of caring. Positive experiences of informal caring on a short-term basis were also reported in a study evaluating hospital at home schemes by Jester & Hicks (2003), as demonstrated in Table 6.2.

It would seem, therefore, that there are a number of explanations as to why informal carers find providing care for a family member a positive experience. Reciprocity, affection, filial obligation and attachment are concepts that have been studied in an effort to explain the initiation and maintenance of caring for a family member (Montenko, 1989). Also, carers may feel more in control of what happens to their relative if they take on the role themselves. They may have negative perceptions of institutional care based on either previous experience or through the media and networking. The presence of formal carers in the patient's own home may be intrusive and disruptive to their daily routines, since care agencies (NHS or independent) are often unable to specify when they will be visiting.

Clearly, there are potential benefits and disadvantages to taking on and maintaining the informal carer role. These need to be honestly discussed with potential carers and revisited at regular intervals throughout the caregiving journey. Failure by us, as specialist practitioners, to recognise that informal carers are not coping can lead to carer strain and burden, with serious consequences for both the health of the carer and the patient.

Carer strain and burden

Longitudinal studies over the last three decades have provided unequivocal evidence that caregiving is stressful (Robinson & Thurnher, 1979; Archbold, 1983). Sources of caregiver stress have been identified and categorised under several subheadings:

- The personal limitations imposed by caregiving
- Competing role demands of the caregiver
- The patient's emotional and physical demands

A large, longitudinal study conducted in the USA by The Select Committee on Aging (1987), found that four types of caregiver strain resulted from the stress of caring: emotional strain; physical strain; financial strain; and family strain.

Carer stress and perceived burden will vary between individuals, depending on the level of support they receive and their own coping strategies. Lazarus & Folkman (1984) developed an interactional theory of stress and coping. This suggests that when an individual is faced with a potential stressor, e.g. caring for a sick and/or dependant relative, they will perform primary and secondary appraisals of the situation: first, to assess if the situation, e.g. caregiving, represents a threat to their well being; and, second, to assess the resources they have at hand to help them to cope with the situation, e.g. level of support from other family members and health care professionals. Carer strain can be experienced by those caring even on a short-term basis, as exemplified by studies evaluating hospital at home schemes. Jester & Hicks (2003) reported that all informal carers said they experienced some degree of burden. There is no evidence in the literature to suggest that carer strain is more evident in either short- or long-term caregiving situations. Miller *et al.* (1997) affirms the complexity of differentiating between the experiences of long- and short-term caregivers, stating: 'There are conflicting findings in the literature as to whether carer stress diminishes or increases with time'. Carer strain is not exclusive to either men or women. Stereotypically, we may assume that female family carers are more willing and able to take on the caregiving role. However, there is no evidence to affirm this assumption. Miller & Cafasso (1992) found that female caregivers reported the role to be a greater burden than male caregivers. An earlier study by Young & Kahana (1989) also found female caregivers to be more negatively affected than males in multiple domains, including greater subjective burden. My own experience affirms that carer stress can be experienced at any point in the caregiver's career irrespective of gender, which reinforces the need for regular and accurate assessment of the informal caregiver's situation.

Measuring carer strain

It is evident from the literature that there has been a tremendous overall lack of consistency in the definitions and measurement of caregiving stress and burden. Robinson (1983) developed the Caregiver Strain Index (CSI), which aims to quantify the degree of strain experienced by informal carers. The categories in the index were derived inductively from a series of open-ended interviews with adult children caring for elderly parents conducted by Robinson in 1979. The index comprises 13 categories, each of which is either scored 1 for yes or 0 for no. The maximum strain score, therefore, would be 13. Robinson (1983) claims that the index has reliability and construct validity for carers of elderly people who have sustained hip fracture, hip replacement or arterio-sclerotic heart disease.

The index has been used extensively in subsequent studies investigating the impact or strain on informal carers. However, as stressed in Chapter 5 any measurement tool must be fit for its purpose, i.e. its psychometric properties must be affirmed. The CSI was validated for administration two months post-hospital discharge, and therefore may be unsuitable for different points in the caregiver's career. Also, the index lacks specificity as the caregiver responses are limited to yes/no answers and participants are unable to quantify or elaborate on the degree or nature of the strain experienced. It is therefore recommended that the CSI be supplemented by the use of a qualitative interview or questionnaire. Because carers should be given the opportunity to express any distress or difficulties in confidence, it is often necessary to arrange to assess the carer away from the patient they are caring for.

The role of specialist nurses in coordinating and leading the support and preparation of informal carers

The first stage is the timely and accurate identification of either an existing or future informal carer. For example, you may receive a new referral for a client requiring case management who has an existing informal carer. An integral part of the initial client assessment should be to identify existing support mechanisms, including the input of informal carers. As discussed earlier in this chapter, the input of informal carers is frequently unknown to health and social services and they may be receiving no support: i.e. have not received any preparation or support for their role. Alternatively, you may identify a potential new informal carer when caring for a client in the early stages of rehabilitation, e.g. on the stroke unit. At this stage it is important to remember that just because a patient has an able relative/friend who can provide care this does not mean that they are willing to do so. Ayling (1993) supports this, recommending: 'do not make assumptions that because carers are present, that they are willing. Do not suppose that all carers and patients have a wonderful relationship. A strained relationship does not suddenly change when a partner becomes a patient.' It requires sensitivity and discretion on behalf of the specialist nurse to ensure family members do not feel coerced into taking on or maintaining the role of informal carer, and that people are given the option of refusal without it resulting in feelings of guilt or conflict with the patient. In addition, it is important to find out if the client is comfortable about their family member or friend taking on the role of carer. The nature of informal caring frequently involves many intimate duties, such as assistance with personal hygiene and toileting, and ones that are physically and emotionally demanding. It is therefore imperative that both the client and the potential informal carer are able to make an informed, uncoerced decision.

If it is established that a family member or friend of the client is willing to take on the role of informal carer and the client supports the proposed action, then the next stage is to establish if their input is going to be required on a short-, medium- or long-term basis and what their role will involve. For example, is the caregiving career predicted to be a short-term one following their relative's early discharge to a hospital at home (HaH) scheme after, for example, a total joint replacement? As having a co-resident family member is often one of the criteria for admission to HaH, it is imperative they are included in the decision-making process regarding early discharge or admission prevention. Sadly, research to date reports that seldom are family members included in the decision-making process (Jester & Hicks, 2003). Or is it a long-term career for a relative with a degenerative condition such as multiple sclerosis?

It is imperative that carers are fully informed about what their role will involve and the predicted length of that commitment, plus honest discussion of the predicted trajectory of their relative's disease process. Individuals may find it difficult to predict if they will be able to cope with the role of informal carer. Several intrinsic and extrinsic factors may help us predict how well an individual will cope with informal caring, including their: locus of control, previous experiences of caregiving situations, coping strategies and level of support from other family members and friends.

Following an informed decision by the relative or friend to take on the informal carer role, their current level of knowledge and experience should be established. One approach to assessing, preparing and educating informal carers is to develop an individualised learning contract. Individual negotiated learning contracts have a number of advantages over standardised training programmes for carers, including:

- Carers and members of the multidisciplinary team develop stronger therapeutic relationships through negotiation of learning contracts.
- Members of the multidisciplinary team develop a better understanding and appreciation of the role of informal carers.
- Learning contracts promote a sense of ownership and responsibility in carers by encouraging them to take control of their learning, and provide them with experience of negotiating and articulating their needs with health care professionals.
- Learning is individualised and builds upon the unique experiences and knowledge of the individual carer.

The first stage in this process is for the carer to self-assess their existing levels of knowledge and experience against identified skills and knowledge. The skills and knowledge required by the informal carer should be developed between the multidisciplinary team and the client. Table 6.3 provides an example of an informal carer individual learning contract. Carers should be supported to assess their level of competence/confidence on a scale ranging from fully competent, partially competent or no prior experience or knowledge. Preparation for the self-management of chronic disease programmes is also highly relevant to informal carers as well as patients themselves. Such preparation focuses on various skills, e.g. problem solving; option appraisal and decision-making; self-efficacy and belief modification; and symptom reinterpretation. (Please refer to Chapter 10 for further detail on preparation for self-management.)

Ongoing support of the informal carer

Following the preparation of the carer to take on their role, the specialist nurse continues to have an important role in the support of the carer. This should include regular assessment of the carer's own needs and early identification of carer strain. Knowledge of the problems of caregivers does not delineate the needs of caregivers. Attention should focus on identifying and describing the needs of caregivers and on designing intervention strategies to meet those needs.

Informal carers deserve respect for their in-depth knowledge of the client's condition and care needs. Many informal carers often report feeling devalued by health professionals, specifically when the patient is admitted to secondary care for investigation or treatment. As specialist nurses we have a pivotal role in ensuring carers are not excluded from the patient's care whilst they are hospitalised and that their expertise is valued. The client and/or carer may reach a point when they can no longer cope and then they will both need support to identify appropriate long-term or palliative residential care. Carers often experience a real loss of purpose and identity if the client moves into care or dies. Informal carer support networks are ideally placed to support the carer through this difficult time.

Conclusions

This chapter has attempted to demonstrate the magnitude of the contribution that informal carers make in the UK, and to present an overview of the role of the specialist nurse and multidisciplinary team in assessing, preparing and supporting informal carers. This is no longer an optional nicety, but a legislative requirement. Many of our rehabilitation clients would be unable to continue to maximise their independence and live at home if it were not for the support, love and dedication of their family and friends.

Table 6.3 An example of an individualised learning contract for preparing informal carers.

Specific skill or knowledge required	Self-assessment of current level of competence/ confidence	Action required to address knowledge/ skill deficit	Responsible person/s
Safe manual handling of the client		Manual handling training for carer, including how to use appropriate aids	Manual handling trainer or physiotherapist
Early detection and prevention of potential complications in the client, e.g. autonomic dysreflexia, pressure sores, deep vein thrombosis or chest infection		Information literature – written/video/ web-based; group or individual teaching session	Specialist/advanced nurse practitioner
Recognising stress in themselves		One-to-one consultation about recognition of stress related to caregiving role and coping strategies. Introduction to CSI	Specialist/advanced nurse practitioner
Knowledge of support mechanisms for carers both in the statutory and voluntary sectors		Provide contact details for local and national support groups. Provision of details of relevant websites	Specialist/advanced nurse practitioner in liaison with link person for support group
Promoting independence in the client		Observation and supervised practice of rehabilitation activities with client	Multidisciplinary team members
Knowledge of their legal rights as a carer		Literature and relevant websites appropriate to carer's educational background	Social worker and specialist/advanced nurse practitioner
Administration of medicines		Explanation of client's medication, including potential side-effects. Safe storage of medication and importance of regular review of medicines by GP/case manager etc.	Pharmacist

References

Archbold P. (1983) Impact of parent-caring on women. *Family Relations*, **32**, 39–45.

Ayling J. (1993) Physiotherapists and carers. *Physiotherapy*, **79**, 780.

Banks P. (1999) *Carer Support: Time for a Change of Direction?* London, King's Fund Publishing.

Cheung J. and Hocking P. (2004) Caring as worrying: the experience of spousal carers. *Journal of Advanced Nursing*, **47** (5), 475–482.

Department of Health (1989) *Caring for People: Community Care in the Next Decade and Beyond*. London, HMSO.

Department of Health (1995) *The Carers (Recognition and Services) Act*. London, The Stationery Office.

Department of Health (2000) *The Carers and Disabled Children Act*. London, The Stationery Office.

Department of Health (2004) *The Carers (Equal Opportunities) Act*. London, The Stationery Office.

Doty R. (1986) Family care of older persons: The role of public policy. *Milbank Memorial Fund Quarterly*, **64**, 34–75.

Griffiths R. (1988) *An Agenda for Action on Community Care*. London, HMSO.

Jarvis A. and Worth A. (2005) The development of a screening tool to identify carers in a general practice by a large-scale mailed survey: the experience in one Scottish general practice. *Journal of Clinical Nursing*, **14**, 363–372.

Jester R. and Hicks C. (2003) Using cost-effectiveness analysis to compare hospital at home and in-patient interventions. Part 1. *Journal of Clinical Nursing*, **12**, 13–19.

Lawton M. (1989) Measuring caregiving appraisal. *Journal of Gerontology: Psychological Sciences*, **44**, 61–71.

Lazarus R. and Folkman S. (1984) *Stress, Appraisal and Coping*. New York, Spring Publishing.

Miller B. and Caffasso L. (1992) Gender differences in caregiving: fact or artefact? *The Gerontologist*, **32**, 498–507.

Miller N., Drummond A. and Jubt L. (1997) Carer health after stroke: the influence of stroke unit treatment. *British Journal of Therapy and Rehabilitation*, **4** (2), 86–90.

Montenko A. (1989) The frustrations, gratifications and well-being of dementia caregivers. *The Gerontologist*, **29**, 263–265.

Powell M. and Kocher P. (1996) *Strategies for Change: A Carer's Impact Resource Book*. London, King's Fund Institute.

Robinson B. (1983) Validation of a Carer Strain Index. *Journal of Gerontology*, **38** (3), 344–348.

Robinson B. and Thurnher M. (1979) Taking care of aged parents: A family cycle transition. *The Gerontologist*, **19**, 583–593.

Rowlands O. and Parker G. (1998) *Informal Carers. Results of an Independent Study Carried Out on Behalf of the Department of Health as Part of the 1995 General Household Survey*. London, The Stationery Office.

Select Committee on Aging (1987) *Exploding the Myths: Caregiving in America*. Washington DC, Government Printing Office, Comm. Pub. NO99–66–11.

Smith L., Lawrence M., Kerr S., Langhorne P. and Lees K. (2004) Informal carers' experience of caring for stroke survivors. *Journal of Advanced Nursing*, **46** (3), 235–244.

Young R. and Kahana E. (1989) Specifying caregiver outcomes: gender and relationship aspects of caregiving strain. *The Gerontologist*, **29**, 660–666.

Chapter 7
Rehabilitation of Orthopaedic Patients

Rebecca Jester

This chapter aims to provide an overview of rehabilitation processes related to both elective orthopaedic conditions and following trauma such as fractures. The indicative content includes:

- Overview of orthopaedic patients requiring rehabilitation.
- Discussions on demography and aetiology.
- The role of the specialist nurse working with patients suffering from osteoarthritis.
- The role of the specialist nurse in falls' prevention and management, together with an update on research-based strategies.
- The role of the specialist nurse working with elderly trauma patients, focusing on femoral neck fracture and other pathological fractures (patient navigator).

Overview of orthopaedic patients requiring rehabilitation

A significant number of orthopaedic and trauma conditions require comprehensive rehabilitation regimens to help patients achieve their maximum independence and quality of life. Many orthopaedic patients are older and suffer with several comorbid states as well as their primary orthopaedic condition. Specialist nurses have an important role in pre-habilitation to prepare patients prior to elective orthopaedic surgery, e.g. total joint replacement, and in rehabilitation following both elective procedures and treatment for fractures and other types of trauma. Within the scope of this chapter the discussion will focus on osteoarthritis and total joint replacement, surgical fixation of hip fractures and the prevention and management of falls. The rationale for the inclusion of these areas is due to the enormity of their prevalence both in the UK and North America. Rehabilitation for all orthopaedic and trauma patients will take place in a variety of settings, including: acute orthopaedic wards; hospital rehabilitation units; community-based schemes, such as Hospital at

Home; and intermediate and step-down facilities (please see Chapter 3 for further details).

Osteoarthritis

Osteoarthritis (OA) is the commonest cause of severe disability among the older population in the UK and in North America (Hosie & Dickson, 2000) and is the biggest cause of joint pain, which provides a major challenge to health care (Jones & Doherty, 1999). It is suggested that 11% of people diagnosed with OA are forced to work reduced hours and 14% to retire early because of their condition (Hosie & Dickson, 2000). Furthermore, OA accounted for over 3 million GP consultations in 2000 (OHE, 2001) and 114 628 hospital admissions (DH, 2000) in the UK. Weight-bearing joints, such as the hip and knee, are most commonly affected and it is quite common for patients to suffer with OA in several joints concurrently leading to severe pain, disability and loss of function.

Despite a wealth of research into the aetiology of OA the exact cause/s remain uncertain. Formerly, it was thought to be a progressive degenerative condition and an inevitable part of the physiological processes of ageing. However, in recent years it has been suggested the disease is a metabolically active process, which affects all joint tissue. Altered biomechanical forces affecting the articular cartilage and subchondral bone, due in part to congenital and/or developmental disease (e.g. congenital hip dysphasia, Perthe's disease) and biochemical changes in the articular cartilage, are important factors in the pathogenesis of OA.

Abnormal load-bearing due to excessive external forces through the joint are also thought to be likely contributors to the disease process. External forces may be attributed to obesity and/or cumulative excessive exposure to overuse, which results in abnormal repetitive strain being placed upon the joint/s. This is exemplified within my own patient caseload with many window cleaners, builders and carpet fitters presenting with severe OA of the knee joint/s. Obesity is a major risk factor for OA of the knee, particularly in middle-aged women, in whom for every 5-kg increase in weight the risk increases by 30% (Jones & Doherty, 1999). Specialist nurses have an important role to play in patient education and in supporting patients to minimise contributory factors through weight loss and lifestyle modification. They also have a public health role, working with health care colleagues, such as school nurses and those responsible for well persons' clinics, to provide education and support for lifestyle modification to prevent or delay the onset of OA.

Signs and symptoms

There is often incongruence between the severity of symptoms reported by patients and the signs visible on X-ray (Nilsdotter, 2001). It is therefore vitally

Table 7.1 Signs and symptoms of osteoarthritis.

Signs
• Crepitus
• Restriction of passive/active range of movement of the joint/s
• Shortening
• Alterations in gait, e.g. Trendelburg flexion and external rotation of the hip and genu varus deformity of the knee
• Radiographic changes: loss of joint space, osteophyte formation, subluxation, subchondral sclerosis and or cysts, spurs at the joint margins
Symptoms
• Pain on movement and at rest, disturbed sleep
• Joint stiffness
• Reduced mobility/function due to pain/deformity/stiffness

important that radiological evidence is not used as an exclusive indication for treatment options. A summary of the clinical features of OA is presented in Table 7.1 and radiological changes are demonstrated in Figs 7.1 and 7.2, which illustrate narrowing of the joint space in a knee joint, particularly on the lateral aspect. Specialist nurses using holistic approaches to assessment and clinical decision-making should focus on the impact of the symptoms on the patient and their coping strategies. Increasingly, pre-habilitation and self-management approaches are being led by specialist nurses in liaison with other members of the multidisciplinary team to support patients with managing their symptoms, either whilst awaiting surgical intervention or as a non-surgical treatment option. Further discussion of these approaches is provided below.

Goals of management

There is no known cure for OA, but thoughtful evidence-based management of the individual patient can reduce their pain, maintain and/or improve joint mobility and limit functional disability. The goals of management of patients with OA are to control pain and other symptoms, minimise disability and educate them and their family about the disease and its therapy.

Before considering therapeutic options in an individual with OA of the hip, it must be certain that the patient's pain is indeed attributable to OA. For instance, it is not infrequent that a patient with a periarticular disorder such as trochanteric bursitis or piriformis syndrome is treated erroneously for hip OA. In addition, it is quite common for joint pain to be referred and patients with disorders of the spine can present with hip pain and those reporting knee pains may have a hip disorder.

Treatment options and the role of the specialist nurse

Treatment options can be broadly classified into conservative and surgical interventions, as summarised in Table 7.2. The specialist nurse has a key role

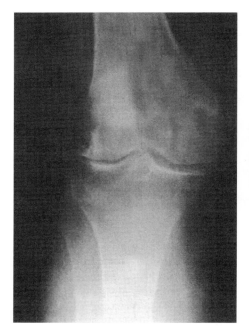

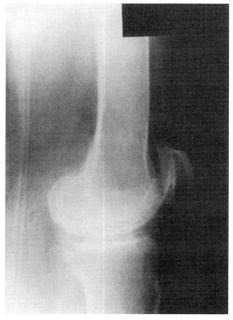

Fig. 7.1 Lateral view of left knee. Reproduced from Jester *et al.* (2005), with kind permission of Churchill Livingstone.

Fig. 7.2 Anterior view of left knee. The joint space is reduced, particularly laterally. Reproduced from Jester *et al.* (2005), with kind permission of Churchill Livingstone.

in empowering patients to make informed choices about which treatment option is appropriate for them at a particular point in time. The principles of rehabilitation are needed whichever of these options is taken.

A significant body of evidence exists to suggest that patients report high levels of satisfaction when many of the conservative treatment options provided in Table 7.2 are led by specialist nurses. Bhattacharyya *et al.* (2005) reported that joint injection clinics led by specialist nurses were an effective means of resource regeneration, with patients reporting fewer complications, reduced injection-site pain and high levels of satisfaction with the service. Flynn (2005) similarly reported high levels of patient satisfaction with specialist nurse-led review clinics following total joint replacement. The specialist nurse can make a significant impact on the quality of outcomes and patient satisfaction throughout many of the treatment options discussed. Patients reported feeling better prepared for their joint replacement surgery when specialist nurses led pre-operative preparation and assessment services (Lucas, 2002).

Increasingly specialist nurses are leading pre-habilitation services prior to patients undergoing procedures such as joint arthroplasty or resurfacing. The

Table 7.2 Treatment options for osteoarthritis.

Conservative options

Patient education, e.g. self-management programmes: individuals who attend these programmes report decreased pain, decreased frequency of physician visits and overall improvement in quality of life. Additional educational materials, including videos, pamphlets and newsletters, are available from the Arthritis Council (ARC).

Weight loss (if overweight): this will reduce weight-bearing load through joints and also encourage the client to engage in exercise regimens to improve muscle strength and tone.

Physical therapy: range of motion and strengthening exercises, assistive devices for ambulation, e.g.: proper use of a stick (in the hand contralateral to the affected joint) reduces the loading forces on the joint and is associated with decreased pain and improved function; and aerobic aquatic exercise programmes.

Occupational therapy: joint protection and energy conservation, assistive devices for activities of daily living.

Assessment and evidence-based management of pain: in recent years concerns about possible deleterious effects of NSAIDs on articular cartilage metabolism and recognition of the greater risk of toxicity from prolonged NSAID therapy in elderly patients negates routine use of NSAIDs in patients with osteoarthritis.

Joint injections using local anaesthetic and/or steroids: provides pain relief through resolution of inflammation in soft tissue. Short-term relief for 2 weeks to 12 months.

Surgical options

Joint resurfacing: an alternative to total joint replacement for younger patients and constitutes a time-buying, first-stage operation.

Osteotomy: performed to reduce the load on the most severely affected part of the joint.

Arthrodesis: surgical fusion of the joint provides pain relief, but the patient has no or very little movement in the joint.

Total joint replacement: removal of the articulating surfaces of the joint and replacement with plastic or metal components.

Autologous Cartilage Transplant (ACT): two-stage procedure, which involves obtaining cartilage cells from a non-weight bearing aspect of the patient's affected knee and transplantation of the cells 4−6 weeks later onto the defective area of the joint.

---

aim of pre-habilitation is often threefold: to teach patients exercises to increase muscle tone and strength; to ensure that any comorbid medical conditions (e.g. hypertension, angina or skin disorders) are monitored and controlled in the pre-operative period; to provide information about the procedure and post-operative regimens to maximise patient concordance and reduce anxiety.

Post-operatively, it is essential that rehabilitation is not viewed in the narrow context of being limited to time spent with the physiotherapists. As discussed in Chapter 2, the carry-on-function of the nurse in rehabilitation is essential to ensure all therapeutic interventions are aimed at successful completion of the agreed rehabilitation goals. Therefore, the specialist nurse must be competent and confident in mobilisation and therapy techniques following procedures such as total joint replacement, including:

- Positioning and movement to minimise the risk of dislocating the hip prosthesis.
- Selecting appropriate walking aids and instructing the patient on their gait using the walking aid/s.
- Appropriate muscle strengthening exercise regimens.
- Instructing the patient on stair safety.
- Measuring active and passive range of joint movements using goniometry.
- Assessing muscle strength and tone.
- Evaluating patients' progress against the identified integrated care pathway.
- Fitting and adjusting relevant modifications and aids such as raised toilet seats, bed and chair blocks, etc.

The specialist nurse, in liaison with the physiotherapist and occupational therapist, has an important role in providing education and training to nursing and support staff caring for patients following procedures such as total joint replacement, both in the hospital and community setting. This involves ensuring that correct mobilisation and exercise regimens are integrated into all aspects of the patients' daily activities and are not simply left to the relatively short periods spent with the physiotherapist. A significant factor in the efficacy of rehabilitation is patients' motivation to actively work toward their rehabilitation goals. The specialist nurse needs to assess the patient's psychological status and knowledge related to their rehabilitation goals and what is expected of them, and to action any knowledge deficits and/or provide psychological support.

One of the key factors of success in rehabilitation following major orthopaedic surgery is effective pain management. It is immoral to expect patients to participate in rehabilitation activities, including mobilisation and exercise regimens, unless their pain is well controlled. Many older people believe pain is inevitable following surgery and frequently underreport their pain to nursing and medical staff. Older people are often also fearful of addiction to analgesia and of side-effects such as constipation, nausea and dizziness. This is frequently compounded by inadequate pain assessment by health care professionals, specifically in patients with cognitive dysfunction. Middleton (2004) suggested the tenets of good management of pain include: regular pain assessment and scoring with a valid tool; believing patients' assessment of their own pain; and administering appropriate drugs in correct doses, at correct intervals via appropriate routes and delivery methods. The specialist nurse has an important role in educating both staff and patients about the importance of effective pain management in rehabilitation, and utilising further expertise, if needed, through specialist pain management teams.

Evidence-based risk management strategies to prevent complications, such as deep vein thrombosis, primary and secondary infection and dislocation of the hip prosthesis, are essential if the patient is to achieve their rehabilitative goals in the agreed timeframe (Jester, 2005).

The role of the specialist nurse in falls' prevention and management

Falls are the leading cause of accidental death in older people, with over 400 000 older people in England attending emergency departments following a fall. In addition, up to 14 000 people a year die in the United Kingdom as a result of an osteoporotic hip fracture (DH, 2001; Legge, 2003). Studies estimating the prevalence of falls in the elderly range from 23% to 59% of older people in hospital or institutional care and between 28% and 60% of older people at home. Almost 50% of falls in hospital occur near the bed (Mosley *et al.*, 1998), with the others occurring in the corridor, bathroom or toilet. There is contraindicatory evidence as to when falls are more likely to occur, some suggest falls are more likely during the early period of admission, possibly because of unfamiliar surroundings (Downton, 1993). However, Stevenson *et al.* (1998) have suggested that falls are more likely to occur during the later stages of rehabilitation as patients' mobility increases.

Falling impacts adversely on older people's morbidity and mortality. Moreover, there are a number of significant negative physical, social and psychological sequels following a fall, including self-imposed restricted mobility, fall phobia and fractures.

The importance of reducing the number of fall-related injuries in the older population has been highlighted by Standard 6 of the National Service Framework for Older People (DH, 2001), which states that providers of health and social care must work together to reduce the number of fall-related injuries occurring within the elderly population. In addition, older people who have fallen should receive effective treatment and rehabilitation and have access to a specialist falls' service.

Although the risk of falling can never be totally eliminated, it can be significantly reduced by using valid methods of assessment and the introduction of falls' prevention strategies (Cannard, 1996; Oliver *et al.*, 1997; Close *et al.*, 1999). Indeed, the very nature of rehabilitation is to maximise independence and this carries an inherent risk of falling. However, this risk needs to be managed through environmental adaptation and the resolution of any intrinsic risk factors, as well as a comprehensive educational programme for staff, patients and carers.

Assessing the risk of falls

Effective assessment of a person's risk of falling requires an understanding of the intrinsic and extrinsic risk factors, a summary of which is provided in

Table 7.3   Intrinsic and extrinsic risk factors of falling.

Intrinsic factors	Extrinsic factors
• Postural hypotension • Altered balance and/or gait • Polypharmacy • Urgency/frequency of micturition • Confusion/cognitive impairment • Loss of muscle tone/mass • Sensory impairment • Previous history of falls	• Ill-fitting footwear • Unfamiliar surroundings • Poor lighting • Loose floor covering • Inappropriate walking aids • Staff to patient ratio • Experience of staff in identifying risk of falling • Lack or failure of equipment

Table 7.3. Also, there is a need to carry out a post-fall assessment, this includes history taking and examination to establish which physiological and environmental factors contributed to the fall.

In response to the need to reduce the risk of falling in the elderly population there has been a proliferation of assessment tools designed to predict patients' risk of falling, including the Fall Risk Assessment Scale for the Elderly (FRASE), St Thomas's Risk Assessment Tool in Falling Elderly Inpatients (STRATIFY) and the Morse Fall Scale (MFS). These tools aim to establish a person's risk of falling based upon the calculation of a number of intrinsic factors associated with falling; however, they generally fail to take into account extrinsic risk factors. As discussed in Chapter 5, it is essential that any assessment tool is valid, reliable, specific, sensitive and practical. Unfortunately, there is little empirical evidence supporting the psychometric properties of falls' risk assessment tools widely used in rehabilitation settings. This has been affirmed by a number of validation studies.

O'Connell & Myers (2002) investigated the predictive accuracy of the MFS and reported the scale had poor sensitivity and specificity, with an 18% positive prediction value. A local validation study and a remote validation study were carried out for STRATIFY, which is based on five factors (Seed *et al.*, 1998). A risk score of two or more had a 'sensitivity of 93% and a specificity of 88%' (Oliver *et al.*, 1997; p. 1051) in the local validation study and a 'sensitivity of 92% and a specificity of 68%' (Oliver *et al.*, 1997; p. 1051) in the remote validation study.

An independent validation of FRASE indicated it is 'effective in predicting the likelihood of falls' (Cannard, 1996; p. 37). Since the introduction of FRASE the number of patients who have fallen has been reduced by 15% and the number of fall incidents have been reduced by 22% (Cannard, 1996). However, the validation study did not specifically examine the sensitivity and specificity of FRASE.

A number of factors prompted the author to undertake a further validation study of both FRASE and STRATIFY, including the lack of research exploring the predictive accuracy of either FRASE or STRATIFY specifically with hip fracture patients. In addition, the interreliability of the two tools has not been proven, and some of the factors included within the tools may be ambiguous and susceptible to a high degree of subjectivity: for example, the term 'agitation' is fairly difficult to differentiate from confusion, dementia or restlessness in the clinical setting. The study reported that inter-rater reliability for both tools was high, but the predictive accuracy of both tools was poor with a propensity for them to overpredict the risk of falling (Jester *et al.*, 2005). It may appear preferable for falls' risk assessment tools to over- rather than underpredict, but, in busy rehabilitation settings it is imperative that finite resources needed to implement falls' prevention strategies are directed at those really at risk. Therefore the use of these tools in isolation is not enough to accurately identify a risk of falling and should be an adjunct to holistic assessment, examination and clinical investigation of the patient.

Falls' prevention strategies

Specialist nurses have a direct responsibility to identify those at risk within their own case loads, and to work with the other members of the multidisciplinary team to ensure all staff working within rehabilitation are able to accurately assess the risk of falling and to implement individualised evidence-based falls' prevention strategies. Failure to do this will severely impact on the rehabilitation process and can lead to patient injury and possible death, as well as the legal implications of potential litigation due to negligence.

Following a comprehensive falls' risk assessment an individualised falls' prevention strategy should be developed in liaison with the patient, their family and other members of the multidisciplinary team. Prevention of falls and minimising the fear of falling should be included in the goal setting phase of the rehabilitation process. Depending on the intrinsic and extrinsic factors identified during the assessment process, appropriate adaptations should be made to the patient's environment, be that in their own home or within an inpatient rehabilitation setting. Careful positioning of support rails, adequate lighting and removal of unnecessary items that may lead to trips are relatively simple adaptations that can be made. Furthermore, the distance to the toilet can be reduced in an inpatient area by ensuring the patient's bed is as near to the toilet as possible, rather than in an end bay, etc. Resolving continence issues may involve referral to the continence specialist if the rehabilitation team are unable to ascertain the cause of incontinence and more detailed clinical investigations are required, such as urodynamics. Comprehensive medicines' review should help to minimise issues related to polypharmacy. When the falls' prevention strategy has been agreed and implemented, it is important that the patient's at-risk status is re-assessed at regular intervals and the efficacy of the falls' prevention strategy evaluated.

The rehabilitation team must address the issue of fear of falling with the patient, as this can often lead to a reluctance to mobilise and to become as independent as possible. One technique used to help patients regain their confidence is to use 'managed falls'. Here, patients are supported and gently lowered to the floor, preferably in their own home environment or one similar to it, and are shown how they can get themselves up after a fall by raising themselves first to their knees using available solid furniture. Many older patients fear falling at home and being unable to summon help quickly and subsequently developing hypothermia. Providing them with personal alarms to wear around their necks and cordless phones to carry in their pockets can alleviate anxiety. Also, having a flask of a hot drink and a blanket near them in the main room they use will ensure that, in the event of a fall, they can keep themselves warm until help arrives. Clearly, this will not remove all risk of hypothermia, but it will reduce it. Hip protectors can also be useful for some patients, as the impact of the fall is dissipated away from the hip and prevents fracture. Low impact and seated exercise classes for older people can help to improve their balance and muscle strength and help to prevent falls.

Hip fracture

Fractured hip is a relatively common occurrence in older people. In 1997/98 it accounted for 66 000 hospital admissions in England and Wales (Audit Commission, 2000), an increase of 10% on the previous year. It is reported that this trend is continuing annually, and rises exponentially with the ageing population. Hip fracture in older people can result from a relatively low impact injury because of poor bone density due to osteoporosis and is often the result of a fall. Mortality rates following hip fracture are high, being estimated to be as high as 40% within the first year following the fall; furthermore, relatively few patients achieve their pre-fracture functional status (Williams & Jester, 2005).

Hip fracture classification and treatment modalities

Hip fractures can be classified into intra- or extracapsular (see Fig. 7.3). Intracapsular fractures can result in damage to the blood supply to the femoral head, leading to delayed or non-union and avascular necrosis of the femoral head. There are two treatment options: undisplaced fractures are reduced and internally fixed; and displaced fractures or pathological fractures should be treated with either total hip replacement or hemiarthroplasty. Extracapsular fractures require internal fixation with dynamic hip screws.

A number of national reports have recommended early surgical repair of the fracture, within 24 hours, to reduce patient mortality and morbidity. However, there is a paucity of empirical evidence supporting a possible link between delayed surgery and post-operative mortality; furthermore, patients presenting with hip fractures are not a homogenous group and the causes of post-operative mortality are multifactorial. Williams & Jester (2005) explored the relationship between time to surgical internal fixation and post-operative mortality using a retrospective correlational design, and found there was no relationship between delayed surgery and post-operative mortality. The study

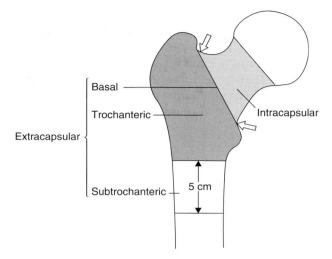

Fig. 7.3 Classification of hip fractures.

reported that post-operative mortality was multifactoral and that cognitive dysfunction and older age were both good prognostic indicators of an increased mortality risk within the first year. Furthermore, it is important that patients are adequately prepared and resuscitated before surgery is carried out.

Rehabilitation of hip fracture patients

Sadly, rehabilitation following hip fracture continues to be fragmented and suboptimal in many areas, resulting in few patients regaining their pre-fracture status. Many trauma and orthopaedic teams continue to view rehabilitation as a place where the patient will be sent to if and when a bed becomes available, rather than a goal directed process that must begin as soon as the patient is medically stabilised and their fracture fixed. It is essential that once the patient has been medically stabilised following internal surgical fixation, and fixation is confirmed by X-ray, mobilisation should, ideally, begin within 24 hours of surgery. Positioning and mobilisation will vary depending on whether the fracture was treated with a dynamic hip screw or a hemi or total prosthesis. As outlined earlier, pain management and the prevention of post-operative complications, such as wound infection, dislocation of the prosthesis, deep vein thrombosis and pressure sores, are essential in order for the patient to be able to actively participate in rehabilitation activities.

It has been long been recognised that hospitalising older people often has a deleterious impact on their physical and psychosocial health. Rehabilitation is often more realistic in the patient's own home, as discussed in Chapter 3. Therefore the specialist nurse in rehabilitation has a pivotal role in expediting a safe and early discharge from the trauma unit, either to the patient's own home or step-down facilities. As it is also important that the integrated pathway for hip fracture patients engenders the principles of early goal directed rehabilitation, the specialist nurse will need to provide support and education to nurses and carers on the acute orthopaedic unit to ensure maximum independence is achieved.

Many orthopaedic medical teams continue to focus solely on the fixation of the hip fracture with little attention paid to preventing further falls and treatment for osteoporosis. As mentioned above, nearly all hip fractures in older people are the result of a relatively low impact injury sustained from a fall, and because of reduced bone density due to osteoporosis they sustain a pathological fracture. Therefore, it is important the specialist nurse ensures that all patients presenting with a hip fracture undergo a comprehensive falls' risk assessment and are referred to specialist falls' services if further expertise is needed. In addition, all patients should be investigated for osteoporosis and be given appropriate pharmacological treatment, such as: bisphosphonates and calcintonin to prevent further loss of bone density. Patients should be assessed on an individual basis to ascertain if hip protectors would be useful in preventing further fractures of the hip.

Conclusions

This chapter has discussed the importance of the specialist nurse's role in liaising with trauma and orthopaedic teams to ensure that rehabilitation is seen as an integral part of the patient's journey, and that the interface between acute orthopaedics and rehabilitation is seamless. Also discussed has been the importance of pre-habilitation prior to elective procedures to maximise patient concordance, understanding and physical status following surgery. The need to critically examine the psychometric properties of falls' risk assessment tools has been highlighted, and it has been recommended these are used as an adjunct to comprehensive holistic patient assessment and post-fall analysis. Finally, the importance of medical stabilisation prior to surgery and early rehabilitation following hip fracture have been discussed.

References

Audit Commission (2000) *United They Stand. Co-ordinating Care for Elderly Patients with Hip Fractures*. Abingdon, Audit Commission Publications.

Bhattacharyya M., Bradley H., Teherani A. and Gerber B. (2005) Nurse practitioner's knee injection clinics in the UK: The patient's perception. *Journal of Orthopaedic Nursing*, **9**, 134–139.

Cannard G. (1996) Falling Trend. *Nursing Times*, **92** (1), 36–37.

Close J., Ellis M., Hooper R., Glucksman E., Jackon S. and Swift C. (1999) Prevention of falls in the elderly trial (PROFET): a randomised controlled trial. *Lancet*, **353**, 93–97.

Department of Health (2000) *Hospital Episode Statistics 1999/2000*. London, DH.

Department of Health (2001) *National Service Framework for Older People*. London, DH.

Downton J. (1993) *Falls in the Elderly*. Kent, Hodder & Stoughton Ltd.

Flynn S. (2005) Nursing effectiveness: An evaluation of patient satisfaction with a nurse led orthopaedic joint replacement review clinic. *Journal of Orthopaedic Nursing*, **9**, 156–165.

Hosie G. and Dickson J. (2000) *Managing Osteoarthritis in Primary Care*. Oxford, Blackwell Science.

Jester R. (2005) Osteoarthritis and total joint replacements. In: *Orthopaedic and Trauma Nursing*, 2nd edn (J. Kneale and P. Davis, eds). Edinburgh, Churchill Livingstone.

Jester R., Wade S. and Henderson K. (2005) A pilot investigation of the efficacy of falls risk assessment tools and prevention strategies in an elderly hip fracture population. *Journal of Orthopaedic Nursing*, **9**, 27–34.

Jones A. and Doherty M. (1999) Osteoarthritis. In: *ABC of Rheumatology* (M.L. Snaith, ed.) London, British Medical Journal Publishing Group, pp. 28–31.

Legge A. (2003) Breaking the fall. *Nursing Times*, **99** (1), 23–25.

Lucas B. (2002) Developing the role of the nurse in the orthopaedic outpatient and pre-admission assessment setting. *Journal of Orthopaedic Nursing*, **6**, 153–160.

Middleton C. (2004) Barriers to the provision of effective pain management. *Nursing Times*, **100** (3), 42–45.

Mosley A., Galindo-Ciocon D., Peak N. and West M. (1998) Initiation and evaluation of a research based fall prevention programme. *Journal of Nursing Care Quality*, **13** (2), 38–44.

Nilsdotter D. (2001) Radiographic stage of OA or sex of the patient does not predict one year outcome after THA. *Annals of the Rheumatic Diseases*, **60**, 228–232.

O'Connell B. and Myers H. (2002) The sensitivity and specificity of the Morse fall scale in an acute care setting. *Journal of Clinical Nursing*, **11**, 134–136.

Office for Health Economics (2001) *Compendium of Health Statistics*. London, OHE.

Oliver D., Briton M., Seed P., Martin F. and Hooper A. (1997) Development and evaluation of evidence based practice risk assessment tool (STRATIFY) to predict falls in elderly people. *British Medical Journal*, **315**, 1049–1053.

Seed P., Oliver D., Martin P. and Hooper A. (1998) Authors defend their study to develop tool to predict falls in elderly people. *British Medical Journal*, **316**, 1318.

Stevenson B., Mills E., Eelin L. and Beal K. (1998) Falls risk factors in an acute care setting: a retrospective study. *Canadian Journal of Nursing Research*, **30** (3), 165–173.

Williams A. and Jester R. (2005) Delayed surgical fixation of fractured hips in older people: impact on mortality. *Journal of Advanced Nursing*, **52** (1), 63–69.

Chapter 8
Stroke Care

Tara Chambers

Introduction

In recent years, an influx of research findings has shaped improvements in the management and care of the stroke patient. Stroke has become increasingly higher on the political agenda, and it may be argued this is as a result of the huge financial burden of stroke on the National Health Service (NHS). Over 4% of NHS costs are spent on stroke care per annum (Royal College of Physicians, 2000). Furthermore, the cost implications of stroke can persist after discharge from hospital, and a considerable amount of social services' budgets are spent on providing continuing care. Developments in acute medical treatments and approaches to stroke rehabilitation continue to gain momentum, and have essentially highlighted the fundamental role the nurse plays in the specialty of stroke medicine.

This chapter will discuss evidence-based practices within the acute and rehabilitation phases of stroke, and consider issues relating to stroke service organisation. In addition, the chapter aims to clarify the role of the nurse in stroke care. The chapter includes discussion of the following:

- Epidemiology of stroke
- Diagnostics
- Stroke service organisation and service provision
- Initial management of stroke in the acute phase
- Stroke rehabilitation services
- The nursing role
- Palliative care

Epidemiology of stroke

Every year in England and Wales, approximately 110 000 people will have their first stroke and approximately 30 000 will have a recurrent event. (DH, 2001). These figures suggest that every five minutes someone new is having a stroke.

Although it is predominately a disease of the older person, the condition can also affect younger people. Risk increases with age and half of cases are people who are 75 years and older. The incidence of stroke in people under 65 years is approximately 27 000 per annum (Rudd *et al.*, 2000). In essence, stroke can affect people of all ages and service provision needs to be directed by this.

Stroke accounts for 10–12% of all deaths in industrialised countries (Wolfe *et al.*, 1996). In the UK, it is the third most common cause of death after heart disease and cancers. Although mortality has declined in recent years, the publication *Saving Lives: Our Healthier Nation* proposes a target to further reduce stroke and heart disease mortality amongst people under 65, by at least a third by the year 2010 (DH, 1999).

Essentially, the introduction of effective antihypertensive agents is one explanation for the decline in stroke mortality. However, improved understanding of the control and management of hypertension and other risk factors has also contributed to this decline. Interestingly, there is lack of evidence to assume that the decrease in stroke mortality must be linked to a decline in incidence. It appears the advances in the management of medical complications following a stroke have contributed to the decrease in mortality rates, although this would not impact on stroke incidence.

Diagnosis of stroke

Definition of stroke

Stroke is defined as 'a clinical syndrome of rapidly developing clinical focal/global signs of loss of cerebral function'. These symptoms last for 24 hours or more, or lead to death, with no apparent cause other than a vascular origin (World Health Organization, 1978).

Focal and non-focal neurological symptoms of stroke

Focal neurological symptoms of stroke are clinical features that arise from a disturbance in an identifiable focal area of the brain (Hankey, 2002). Examples of focal neurological symptoms are unilateral weakness, unilateral altered sensation, or speech disorder (Table 8.1). The clinical features are attributable to focal cerebral ischaemia or haemorrhage.

Non-focal neurological symptoms are not anatomically localising, examples being dizziness or generalised weakness (Table 8.2). Consequently, non-focal symptoms do not always indicate stroke as they are rarely a result of focal cerebral ischaemia or haemorrhage (Hankey, 2002).

Types of stroke

Symptoms of stroke occur as a direct result of a disturbance to the blood supply in the brain. Stroke can be classified into three principal types:

Table 8.1   Focal neurological and ocular symptoms (Hankey, 2002).

Motor symptoms
- Weakness or clumsiness on one side of the body, in whole or in part (hemiparesis)
- Simultaneous bilateral weakness (paraparesis, quadriparesis)*
- Difficulty in swallowing (dysphagia)*
- Imbalance (ataxia)*

Speech/language disturbances
- Difficulty understanding or expressing spoken language (dysphasia)
- Difficulty reading (dyslexia) or writing (dysgraphia)
- Difficulty calculating (dyscalculia)
- Slurred speech (dysarthria)*

Sensory symptoms
Somatosensory
- Altered feeling on one side of the body, in whole or in part (hemisensory disturbance)

Visual
- Loss of vision in one eye, in whole or in part (transient monocular blindness or amaurosis fugax)
- Loss of vision in the left or the right half or quarter of the visual field (hemianopia, quadranopia)
- Bilateral blindness
- Double vision (diplopia)*

Vestibular symptoms
- Spinning sensation (vertigo)*

Behavioural or cognitive symptoms
- Difficulty dressing, combing hair, cleaning teeth, etc.; geographical disorientation; difficulty copying diagrams such as a clock (visual–spatial–perceptual dysfunction)
- Forgetfulness (amnesia)*

*As an isolated symptom, this does not necessarily indicate transient focal ischaemia, because there are many other potential causes.

Table 8.2   Non-focal neurological symptoms (Hankey, 2002).

Generalised weakness and/or sensory disturbance
Light-headedness
Faintness
'Blackouts' with altered or loss of consciousness or fainting, with or without impaired vision in both eyes
Incontinence of urine and faeces
Confusion
Any of the following symptoms, if isolated*

- spinning sensation (vertigo)
- ringing in the ears (tinnitus)
- difficulty in swallowing (dysphagia)
- slurred speech (dysarthria)
- double vision (diplopia)
- loss of balance (ataxia)

*If these symptoms occur in combination, or with focal neurological symptoms, they may indicate focal cerebral ischaemia.

- Ischaemic stroke
- Primary intracerebral haemorrhage
- Subarachnoid haemorrhage

The most common type is an ischaemic stroke, otherwise known as a 'cerebral infarction', and accounts for 69% of all strokes (DH, 2001). The cause of a cerebral infarction is decreased blood supply to a specific part of the brain due to obstruction of one of the major cerebral arteries (middle, posterior and anterior) or their smaller perforating branches to deeper parts of the brain. Obstruction of the cerebral blood vessel is a consequence of thrombosis or embolism associated with disease of the blood, blood vessels or heart. A subclassification of cerebral infarctions has been developed, known as the 'Oxfordshire Community Project Stroke Sub Classification' (Bamford *et al.*, 1991; Table 8.3). It is based on areas of anatomical involvement and identifies the subgroups:

- Total anterior circulation infarct
- Partial anterior circulation infarct
- Posterior circulation infarct
- Lacunar infarct

Significant differences in mortality rate and independent functional outcome have been recognised for these subclassifications of cerebral infarctions, and provide a useful tool in suggesting the patient's prognosis and long-term outcome.

A primary intracerebral haemorrhage occurs when a blood vessel bursts causing bleeding into the brain; a subarachnoid haemorrhage is bleeding into the subarachnoid space. Primary intracerebral haemorrhages account for 13% of all strokes, while 6% are due to subarachnoid haemorrhages. Of the remaining strokes, 12% are classified as uncertain in origin (Wolfe *et al.*, 2002).

Initial medical management of the suspected stroke patient is primarily aimed at distinguishing whether the symptoms are due to a vascular event or another cause of neurological disorder with rapid onset. Information on which to base a diagnosis is gathered through comprehensive neurological and systemic assessment and brain imaging.

Brain imaging

Brain imaging, through computed tomography (CT) or magnetic resonance imaging (MRI) scanning of the brain, is used in confirming the diagnosis of stroke. Patients with suspected stroke should have access to CT scanning of the brain within 24 hours of the event (Royal College of Physicians, 2004). Primarily, the purpose of early CT scanning of the brain is to exclude a haemorrhagic stroke and other causes of the symptoms other than stroke (Keir *et al.*, 2002). However, early CT brain scanning will not always detect ischaemic

Table 8.3 The Oxford Community Project Stroke Subclassification (Bamford *et al.*, 1991).

Total anterior circulation infarct (TACI)
Implies a large cortical stroke in the middle cerebral, or middle and anterior cerebral territories. TACI is a combination of:
1. New higher cerebral dysfunction (e.g. dysphasia, dyscalulia, visuospatial disorder)
   AND
2. Homonymous visual field defect
   AND
3. An ipsilateral motor and/or sensory deficit involving at least two out of three areas of the face, arm or leg

Partial anterior circulation infarct (PACI)
Implies cortical stroke in the middle or anterior cerebral artery territory. PACI is:
1. Patient with two out of three components of the TACI
   OR
2. New higher cerebral dysfunction alone
   OR
3. Motor/sensory deficit more restricted than those classified as a LACI

Lacunar infarct (LACI)
Implies a subcortical stroke due to small-vessel disease. LACI is:
1. Pure motor stroke
   OR
2. Pure sensory stroke
   OR
3. Sensorimotor stroke
   OR
4. Ataxic hemiparesis

NB: Evidence of higher cortical involvement or disturbance of conscious level excludes a LACI

Posterior circulation infarct (POCI)
1. Ipsilateral cranial nerve palsy with contralateral motor and/or sensory deficit
   OR
2. Bilateral motor and/or sensory deficit
   OR
3. Disorder of conjugate eye movement
   OR
4. Cerebellar dysfunction without ipsilateral long tract involvement
   OR
5. Isolated homonymous visual field defect

---

stroke. It is estimated that indicators of cerebral infarct are only detected on early CT findings in approximately 50% of cases (Von Kummer *et al.*, 1997).

Urgent brain imaging should be performed if:

- The patient's conscious level is deteriorating
- There is an unexplained fluctuation in medical condition
- Trauma is likely
- The patient has a severe headache on onset of symptoms
- Hydrocephalus secondary to primary intracerebral haemorrhage is suspected

- Neurological diagnosis other than stroke is suspected
- The patient has a history of bleeding or is on anticoagulation therapy (Royal College of Physicians, 2004)

Stroke service organisation and service provision

Stroke units

The National Service Framework for Older People advocates that stroke services should be offered by a specialist stroke team on a designated stroke unit (DH, 2001). Internationally, delivery of organised stroke care has varied. Methods include: acute stroke units; stroke rehabilitation units; or combined stroke units. At present, the evidence to support one method above another in the delivery of care is inconclusive (Dennis & Langhorne, 1994). However, there is unequivocal evidence to affirm that stroke units are effective in reducing mortality by up to 28%, reducing length of hospital stay and institutionalisation (Langhorne *et al.*, 1993). In addition, there is some evidence to suggest stroke unit care can improve functional performance of the patient compared with conventional care (The Stroke Unit Trialists' Collaboration, 1997). Drummond *et al.* (1996) have supported this observation by concluding that stroke unit care significantly improves feeding, dressing and household abilities compared with conventional rehabilitation.

Fundamentally, a stroke unit is a geographically identified unit, with a coordinated multidisciplinary team who are interested and knowledgeable about stroke and rehabilitation (Royal College of Physicians, 2004). The differences between a stroke unit and other hospital wards appear to be organised care systems, the disease-specific interest of staff and the multidisciplinary approach to care. Langhorne (1997) further suggests that additional aspects of stroke units include involving carers in the rehabilitation process and the provision of education and training for staff, patients and carers.

There is little written evidence to indicate what actually constitutes a stroke unit, in terms of the process of rehabilitation. Findings of one study demonstrate that stroke units tend to have: multidisciplinary philosophies, policies and procedures; blanket referral systems to therapy staff; and ward-based multidisciplinary teams (Edman, 2001).

Stroke rehabilitation in the community

Stroke unit care is the favoured model of service organisation, as early, expert and intensive rehabilitation in a hospital stroke unit improves patients' long-term outcome (DH, 2001). However, there will be some incidences where the stroke patient will not be admitted to hospital. Reasons for this include refusal by the individual, or perhaps the diagnosis of stroke would make no difference to management.

Stroke services should be available in the community to aid in supporting early hospital discharge. Nevertheless, early hospital discharge should only be undertaken if there is a specialist stroke rehabilitation team in the community and the patient is able to transfer from bed to chair safely (Early Supported Discharge Trialists, 2005). Consequently, non-specialist or generic rehabilitation teams should not support early hospital discharge of the stroke patient.

Initial management of acute stroke

Depending on the severity of the stroke, there can be an early period (a few days) of spontaneous recovery due to pathophysiological responses aiding in neurological improvement (Hankey, 2002). Spontaneous recovery can account for some improvements during the initial phase, however, this needs to be accompanied by effective acute stroke management and rehabilitation to ensure optimal patient recovery.

Initial screening and monitoring

Stroke is deemed to be a medical emergency. Effective monitoring and treatment in the initial phase after the onset of stroke can reduce the mortality rate and enhance patients' functional outcomes (Royal College of Physicians, 2004). The nurse plays an essential role in the preliminary management of acute stroke. On admission to hospital, the nurse is responsible for assessing the patient's physical and functional ability, including their cognitive state. The patient should receive a formal swallow assessment/screen to ascertain safety of swallow. Special attention is required in relation to the moving and handling needs of the patient (Royal College of Nursing, 2002). In addition, assessment of the patient's skin integrity is vital. The risk of developing pressure sores needs to be screened and documented and appropriate action taken to reduce the risk (National Institute for Clinical Excellence, 2001). As with all assessments, the assessment tools must be reliable and validated, and the choice of measure needs to be clarified at local level.

Fundamental initial care performed by the nurse involves vigilant monitoring of:

- Conscious level
- Temperature
- Blood pressure
- Pulse
- Respirations
- Heart rhythm
- Blood glucose
- Oxygen saturations
- Hydration

Patients with an altered conscious level require close neurological observation, and the most widely used assessment tool for patients with altered levels of consciousness is the Glasgow Coma Scale. In conjunction with neurological observations, vital observations need to be measured. Hypertension is often discovered in the acute post-stroke phase. Monitoring is crucial to detect the need for acute medical treatment of hypertension. Blood pressure should be monitored to ascertain whether it lowers spontaneously or whether intervention is required.

Research examining the choice of arm when measuring blood pressure specifies there is no reason to exclude a hemiplegic upper limb. No noticeable difference between the hemiplegic and unaffected arm has been identified (Panayiotou *et al.*, 1993). Effective practice involves an initial blood pressure check of both arms as differing readings can be obtained, although this is unconnected to the stroke side (Warlow *et al.*, 2001). Further blood pressure measurements should be recorded on the arm with the higher reading.

Essentially, the main reasons for high blood pressure include:

● Direct result of the acute stroke (Fotherby *et al.*, 1993)
● Anxiety due to the event
● Chronic hypertension prior to the stroke (Hankey, 2002)

Throughout the years, there has been much debate about the timely use of antihypertensive agents in the acute phase following a stroke. Aggressive lowering of blood pressure at this stage may result in compromised cerebral perfusion and cerebral blood flow. Most recent evidence indicates that blood pressure should only be lowered in the acute phase, when accelerated hypertension could cause further medical complications such as hypertensive encephalopathy or aortic aneurysm with renal failure (Royal College of Physicians, 2004).

Blood pressure tends to reduce over the first two weeks post-stroke (Warlow *et al.*, 2001). Unless the patient has accelerated blood pressure, antihypertensive agents are commenced at least one to two weeks after the event as a secondary prevention measure (Lindley *et al.*, 1995). Presently, the recommended approach to reducing blood pressure is a thiazide diuretic or an angiotensin-converting enzyme (ACE) inhibitor, or preferably a combination of both unless contraindicated (HOPE, 2000; PROGRESS, 2001). The British Hypertension Society guidelines recommend an optimal blood pressure below 140/85 mmHg and 130/80 mmHg in diabetics (Williams *et al.*, 2004).

Initial treatment of acute ischaemic stroke

Initial medical treatment for an ischaemic stroke is to administer aspirin 300 mg as soon as possible to the onset of the cerebral infarction (Chen *et al.*, 2000). Subsequently, antiplatelet therapy should continue, with the choice of agent being evidence-based and clarified at local level. Thrombolysis is advocated as a potential treatment for cerebral infarction (Royal College of Physicians, 2004). The purpose of thrombolysis is to restore blood flow and reperfuse the ischaemic brain as soon as possible after the cerebral vessel has been occluded. The core of dead brain is surrounded by an area known as the 'penumbra'. It is the penumbra that may be preserved through early intervention with thrombolysis, thus preventing further decline in blood flow. Consequently, thrombolysis may reduce the volume of brain damaged by the cerebral infarct, reduce cerebral oedema and improve clinical outcome (Warlow *et al.*, 2001). Presently, thrombolysis is only being administered by appropriately trained clinicians in hospitals with the equipment to enable effective investigation and monitoring.

Thrombolysis as a viable treatment for patients with ischaemic stroke requires strict controls and its use is only appropriate for highly selected patients. Evidence suggests the window of opportunity from the onset of stroke to the administration of thrombolysis is three hours (ATLANTIS, ECASS and NINDS r-tPA Study Group Investigators, 2004). Although this treatment intervention may increase mortality, it may reduce disability in survivors (Wardlaw *et al.*, 2004).

Initial treatment of primary intracerebral haemorrhage

At present, there is a lack of evidence to suggest that all primary intracerebral haemorrhages would benefit from routine surgical evacuation. However, surgical intervention should be considered for supratentorial haemorrhage with mass effect or a posterior fossa/cerebellar haematoma (Royal College of Physicians, 2004).

Initial treatment of subarachnoid haemorrhage

Primarily, the aim of clinical management of a subarachnoid haemorrhage is to prevent re-bleeding and reduce the risk of secondary complications such as hydrocephalus or cerebral ischaemia. Advice from a neurosurgeon should be sought immediately a diagnosis of subarachnoid haemorrhage has been made (Royal College of Physicians, 2004). Processes need to be in place at the local level to ensure direct and swift access to neurosurgical opinion.

Stroke rehabilitation

The fundamental intentions of treatment and care following a stroke are to:

- Optimise the patient's chance of surviving
- Minimise the impact of the stroke on the patient and carer (Warlow *et al.*, 2001).

The initial management of the acute stroke is concerned with optimising the patient's chance of survival, whereas the principles of rehabilitation are to minimise the impact of stroke on the individual and carer. Standard Five of the *National Service Framework for Older People* reiterates the prompt initiation of rehabilitation following a stroke, and advocates a coordinated approach by a specialist stroke team with expertise in rehabilitation (DH, 2001). Early rehabilitation not only reduces mortality, but has a positive impact on the patient's functional outcome. In addition, early rehabilitation reduces the incidence of discharge to long-term care (The Stroke Unit Trialists' Collaboration, 2001). Hence, difficulties arise when trying to separate the acute and rehabilitation phases of stroke care, as the boundaries of acute care and rehabilitation are obscure and should be viewed as a seamless process. Thus, stroke management needs to adopt an integrated approach. Stroke causes neurological disorganisation, therefore subsequent functional recovery is based on neurological reorganisation. To understand the concept of stroke rehabilitation, it is necessary to briefly discuss how neurological reorganisation is achieved.

Neuromuscular plasticity

Functional recovery following a stroke can occur as intact areas of the brain compensate and take on functions of the damaged area. The reorganisation of connections within the brain is acknowledged as 'plasticity'. Plasticity is the ability of cells to alter any aspect of their phenotype (the physical, biochemical and physiological attributes determined genetically and environmentally), at any stage in their development, in response to abnormal changes (intracellular or extracellular) in their state or environment (Brown and Hardman, 1987). Evidently, restructuring cannot proceed if the whole of the cell body has been destroyed. Consequently, plasticity is concerned with the basis of all neural control, and changing neural activity can be intentionally influenced through clinical rehabilitation. Through repetition of effective rehabilitation activities, positive change can be produced, which, in turn, allows the possibility of restructuring normal movement. To minimise the impact of stroke, rehabilitation needs to commence immediately on diagnosis in order to aid in the principles of neuromuscular plasticity, and to help prevent further complications.

Altered functional ability following a stroke is due to:

- Cognitive and perceptual impairment
- Sensory and motor impoverishment
- Uninhibited reflex activity
- Altered tonicity (Laidler, 2000)

Uninhibited reflex activity and altered tonicity when managed incorrectly can cause problems in recovery, therefore it is essential for the specialist stroke team to adopt an approach that aids in the concept of neuromuscular plasticity.

Therapeutic approach to stroke rehabilitation

To understand the ethos on which rehabilitation is based, the World Health Organization (WHO, 1980) established the International Classification of Disease

(ICD) by identifying impairment, disability and handicap as the key components on which to consider a health condition such as stroke. Yet, in more recent years, the International Classification of Functioning has emerged as the favoured method of explaining the impact of a health condition on the individual, as it suggests a more positive experience for the patient (WHO, 2001). This classification is based on a holistic functional approach and incorporates the effect of a health condition on quality of life. The full range of functional activities that require assessment are:

- Learning and applying knowledge
- General tasks and demands
- Communication
- Mobility
- Self-care domestic life
- Interpersonal interactions
- Major life
- Community, social and civic life

When minimising the impact of stroke on the patient and their family, consideration needs to be given to the effects of the clinical symptoms of the stroke on these identified functional activities. It is essential to deliberate the functional ability of the patient at a physical, psychological and social level, with emphasis on quality of life. Every patient has inimitable needs, so subsequently requires a comprehensive assessment to ascertain their individualised rehabilitation programme through a goal-orientated approach.

Efficacy of stroke rehabilitation

In an early analysis of the efficacy of rehabilitation after stroke, some researchers argued that there was a lack of evidence to support the therapeutic usefulness of stroke rehabilitation, and that functional improvement was due to spontaneous recovery, rather than therapy (Dobkin, 1989). In more recent years, evidence has emerged to support the positive impact that stroke rehabilitation has on functional performance. The evidence is based on research findings which evaluate the effects of different intensities of therapy in stroke rehabilitation. Langhorne *et al.* (1996) conducted a meta-analysis of seven randomised controlled trials of physiotherapy after stroke, and suggested that more physiotherapy input is associated with a reduction in death and improvements in activities of daily living. Most of the randomised controlled trials exploring the effects of different intensities of therapy in stroke rehabilitation have been conducted by physiotherapists. There is a limited amount of evidence from other therapy disciplines. However, a review by Kwakkel *et al.* (1997) critically analysed the results of existing randomised controlled trials to evaluate the effects of different intensities of physiotherapy and occupational therapy input. Results indicate improvements to functional outcome. Based on the available evidence, the Royal College of Physicians (2004) advocated that stroke patients should be seen by relevant therapists and should receive as much therapy as can be tolerated. In addition, patients should be given as much opportunity as possible to practise various skills. More research into minimum thresholds of therapy input is required to enable further advances in the delivery of effective stroke rehabilitation.

In stroke rehabilitation, patients should be offered an optimal learning environment, to enable therapeutic activities to be practised. At present, many differing models of service are offered to provide stroke rehabilitation. However, all models of service should be staffed by specialist experts in stroke and rehabilitation. A geographically identified unit should act as a base, and as part of the inpatient service. However, after the acute phase, specialist stroke services can be effectively delivered to patients in the community, provided that the patient can transfer from bed to chair before going home (Royal College of Physicians, 2004). Where stroke rehabilitation is to occur depends on a number of influential factors, including provision of services, severity of stroke symptoms, medical stability and patients' choice.

The role of the nurse in stroke rehabilitation

Stroke is the main cause of adult disability in the UK, emphasising the importance of effective rehabilitation to aid the patient in reaching their optimum level of independence. Stroke rehabilitation nursing aims to:

- Aid physical recovery from stroke
- Facilitate independence in activities of daily living
- Reduce the risk of secondary complications and related conditions
- Promote holistic adaptation to stroke related disability

Nolan *et al.* (1997) formulated a description of the role of the rehabilitation nurse, based on a systematic review of relevant evidence. While the review was not specific to stroke rehabilitation, the five domains of clinical practice identified are similar to that found in the literature on the nurse's role in stroke care (O'Connor, 1996; Nolan & Nolan, 1998). The identified domains are:

- Promoting physical well being.
- Specialist role in skin care.
- Specialist role in continence.
- A 24-hour presence with the patient, creating and sustaining an environment for rehabilitation and reinforcing the input of other professionals.

Controversially, Burton (2000) suggested that this description actually identifies areas in which rehabilitation nurses can develop, rather than identifying the role itself. Burton (2000), using a reflective enquiry approach, identified three categories of the nursing role in stroke rehabilitation: the nurse as caregiver; facilitator of personal recovery; and care manager. Focusing on the nurse as care manager, this aspect of the nursing role involved liaising, mediating and organising with other members of the multidisciplinary team. The role of care manager in stroke rehabilitation nursing is discussed below and applied in further detail.

Referral to members of the stroke team

To assist the patient in reaching their optimal level, the nurse is responsible for identifying other members of the multidisciplinary team who need to be involved in the patient's care. Essentially, the nurse plays a coordinating role by initiating early referral to other members of the multidisciplinary stroke team. Aims of rehabilitation are best achieved using a multidisciplinary team approach: utilising the resources of several health care professionals as this aids in better functional outcome (The Stroke Unit Trialists' Collaboration, 2001). Nurses are often the most appropriate health care professionals to act in this coordinating role as they develop close therapeutic relationships with patients and their families and are able to provide information relating to the patients' general health, coping and emotional health (Burton, 2000). The type of referral activity relevant to many stroke patients is listed below:

- *Physiological needs* – referral to the speech and language therapist for assessment of swallowing and the dietician for nutritional assessment and dietary planning to maximise energy whilst maintaining safety with swallowing. Referral to the physiotherapist for assessment of mobility, gait and balance and planning of exercise and mobility regimens to maximise muscle strength and tone, minimise the risk of falling and develop optimum manual handling approaches to avoid injury.
- *Social needs* – referral to the occupational therapist for assessment and potential adjustment to the patient's home environment to maximise independence. Referral to social services for support services at home, informal carer support and financial information.
- *Psychological support* – referral to the clinical psychologist when the patient and/or their family have higher level psychological support needs (Levels 3 and 4; see Chapter 4).

Also, the advancing role of the nurse in stroke rehabilitation will increasingly involve liaison with community matrons/case managers; specifically, as many stroke patients will have several comorbid conditions and will meet the criteria for case management. This is not meant to be an exhaustive list of which members of the multidisciplinary team the stroke patient may need referral to, but rather an example of the types of professionals needed to maximise the rehabilitation potential of the patient and to support their family.

Practising therapeutic activities

The National Service Framework for Older People recommends that patients have access to relevant therapists and that each patient is given ample opportunity to practise what is learnt in therapy sessions (DH, 2001). One of the primary roles of the stroke rehabilitation nurse is to assist patients to translate skills learnt in therapy into meaningful activities (Kirkevold, 1997). In essence, nurses are with the patient 24 hours a day, therefore are ideally positioned to sustain the practising of therapeutic activities with the individual patient. However, a study by Booth *et al.* (2001) to compare interventions by nurses and occupational therapists in a stroke unit, implied that occupational therapists use facilitating techniques while nurses tend to 'do for' the patient. This study highlighted the potential discrepancies in consistency in approach to stroke rehabilitation. Stroke rehabilitation nurses require adequate training in how their role can facilitate patient participation in unstructured therapeutic activities. A quasi-experimental study by Booth *et al.* (2005) reported that, following 7 hours of education for nurses working within an inpatient stroke unit focusing specifically on therapeutic handling of stroke patients, the proportion of 'doing for' patient interventions was significantly reduced and facilitatory interventions increased. This suggests that, even with relatively modest educational input, the specific therapeutic role of nurses in stroke rehabilitation can be increased.

Fundamentally, stroke rehabilitation is concerned with practising activities, as this aids positive neuromuscular plasticity and recovery. One may argue it is the role of the nurse to assist patients to translate skills learnt in therapy into meaningful activities, however all members of the multidisciplinary team have a responsibility. All health care members of the specialist stroke team need to share the same philosophy and be involved in practising and repeating activities, as this will help direct an individualised functional approach to the patient's stroke rehabilitation programme.

Reducing the risk of complications

It is paramount that the nurse contributes to reducing the risk of complications following a stroke. Correct positioning is vital in minimising the risk of complications, such as aspiration, respiratory complications, shoulder pain, contractures and pressure sores (Lincoln *et al.*, 1996; National Institute for Clinical Excellence, 2001). A further complication following a stroke is venous thromboembolism, most often found in immobile patients with hemiplegia of the lower limbs. Evidence suggests that deep vein thrombosis can occur in up to 50% of patients with hemiplegia (Warlow *et al.*, 2001). Currently, research findings to suggest the incidence of pulmonary embolism are inconclusive. To aid in reducing the risk of venous thromboembolism, compression stockings should worn by stroke patients with weak or paralysed legs (Amaragiri & Lees, 2000). Further management to reduce the risk includes early mobilisation and optimal hydration (Royal College of Physicians, 2004).

Palliative care

Once it is felt that the patient will not survive, palliative care principles need to be implemented. The stroke nurse requires adequate training in caring for the dying patient to enable effective management of potential symptoms. These include pain, depression, confusion, agitation and problems with hydration and nutrition. In addition, access to palliative care expertise should be available to support in symptom control (National Institute for Clinical Excellence, 2004). The involvement and support of carers is paramount, and carers should be an integral part of the clinical decision-making process.

Conclusions

This chapter has attempted to provide an overview of the magnitude of the impact of stroke on the individual, their family and society as a whole. Evidence-based approaches to the diagnosis and treatment of stroke have emphasised the importance of commencing rehabilitation as soon as possible after stroke, and that patient outcomes are best achieved within a specialist stroke unit.

References

Amaragiri S.V. and Lees T.A. (2000) Elastic compression stockings for prevention of deep vein thrombosis. *The Cochrane Database of Systematic Reviews*, Issue 1. Art No.: CD001484. DOI: 10.1002/14651858. CD001484. http://www.cochrane.org/

ATLANTIS, ECASS and NINDS r-tPA Study Group Investigators (2004) Association of outcome with early stroke treatment: pooled analysis of ATLANTIS, ECASS and NINDS r-tPA stroke trials. *Lancet*, **363**, 768–774.

Bamford J., Sandercock P., Dennis M., Burns J. and Warlow C. (1991) Classification and natural history of clinically identifiable subtypes of cerebral infarction. *Lancet*, **337**, 1521–1526.

Booth J., Davidson I., Winstanley J. and Waters K. (2001) Observing washing and dressing of stroke patients: nursing intervention compared with occupational therapists. What is different? *Journal of Advanced Nursing*, **33** (1), 98–105.

Booth J., Hillier V., Waters K. and Davidson I. (2005) Effects of a stroke rehabilitation programme for nurses. *Journal of Advanced Nursing*, **49** (5), 465–473.

Brown M.A. and Hardman V.J. (1987) Plasticity of vertebrate mononeurons. In: *Growth and Plasticity of Neural Connections* (W. Winslow and C. McCrohan, eds). Manchester, Manchester University Press, pp. 36–51.

Burton C.R. (2000) A description of the nursing role in stroke rehabilitation. *Journal of Advanced Nursing*, **32** (1), 174–181.

Chen Z., Sandercock P., Pan H., *et al.* (2000) Indicators for early aspirin use in acute ischaemic stroke: a combined analysis of 4000 randomized patients from the Chinese Acute Stroke Trial and International Stroke Trial. *Stroke*, **31**, 1240–1249.

Dennis M. and Langhorne P. (1994) So stroke units save lives: where do we go from here? *British Medical Journal*, **309**, 1273–1277.

Department of Health (1999) *Saving Lives: Our Healthier Nation White Paper and Reducing Health Inequalities: An Action Report*. London, NHS Executive.

Department of Health (2001) *National Service Framework for Older People*. London, DH.

Dobkin B.H. (1989) Focused stroke rehabilitation programmes do not improve outcome. *Archives of Neurology*, **41**, 701–703.

Drummond A.E.R., Miller N., Colquohoun M. and Logan P.C. (1996) The effects of a stroke unit on activities of daily living. *Clinical Rehabilitation*, **10**, 12–22.

Early Supported Discharge Trialists (2005) Services for reducing duration of hospital care for acute stroke patients. *The Cochrane Database of Systematic Reviews*, Issue 2. Art No.: CD000443. DOI: 10.1002/14651858. CD000443. pub2. http://www.cochrane.org/

Edman J. (2001) What makes a stroke unit effective? *British Journal of Therapy and Rehabilitation*, **8** (2), 74–77.

Fotherby M.D., Potter J.F., Panayiotou B. and Harper G. (1993) Blood pressure changes after stroke: abolishing the white coat effect. *Stroke*, **24**, 1422.

Hankey G.J. (2002) *Your Questions Answered. Stroke*. London, Churchill Livingstone.

Heart Outcomes Prevention Evaluation Study Investigators (HOPE) (2000) Effects of ramipril on cardiovascular and microvascular outcomes in people with diabetes mellitus: results of the HOPE study and MICRO–HOPE substudy. *Lancet*, **3555**, 253–259.

Keir S., Wardlaw J. and Warlow C. (2002) Stroke epidemiology studies have underestimated the frequency of intracerebral haemorrhage. A systematic review of imaging in epidemiological studies. *Journal of Neurology*, **249**, 1226–1231.

Kirkevold M. (1997) The role of nursing in the rehabilitation of acute stroke patients. *Advances in Nursing Science*, **19**, 55–64.

Kwakkel G., Wagenarr R.C. and Koelman T.W. (1997) Effects of intensity of rehabilitation after stroke: research synthesis. *Stroke*, **28**, 1550–1556.

Laidler P. (2000) Enable or disable: evidence-based clinical problem-solving. In: *Stroke Rehabilitation. A Collaborative Approach* (R. Fawcus, ed.). Oxford, Blackwell Science, pp. 55–82.

Langhorne P. (1997) The stroke unit story. *Stroke Matters*, **1** (2), 1.

Langhorne P., Williams B.O., Gilchrist W. and Howie K. (1993) Do stroke units save lives? *Lancet*, **342**, 395–397.

Langhorne P., Wagenarr R.C. and Partridge C. (1996) Physiotherapy after stroke: more is better? *Physiotherapy Research International*, **1**, 75–88.

Lincoln N.B., Willis D., Phillips S.A., Juby L.C. and Berman P. (1996) Comparisons of rehabilitation practice on hospital wards for stroke patients. *Stroke*, **27**, 18–20.

Lindley R.I., Amayo E.O. and Marshall J. (1995) Hospital services for patients with acute stroke in the United Kingdom. *Age and Ageing*, **24**, 525–532.

Mohr J.P., Biller J., Hilal S.K., *et al.* (1995) Magnetic resonance versus computed tomographic imaging in acute stroke. *Stroke*, **26**, 807–812.

National Institute for Clinical Excellence (2001) *Pressure ulcers – risk assessment and prevention (Guideline B)*. London, NICE.

National Institute for Clinical Excellence (2004) *Supportive and palliative care for people with cancer: Part A and Part B*. London, NICE.

Nolan M. and Nolan J. (1998) Stroke 2: expanding the nurse's role in stroke rehabilitation. *British Journal of Nursing*, **7** (7), 388–393.

Nolan M., Booth A. and Nolan J. (1997) *New Directions in Rehabilitation: Exploring the Nursing Contribution (Research Report Series Number 6)*. London, English National Board for Nursing, Midwifery and Health Visiting.

O'Connor S. (1996) Stroke units: centres of nursing innovation. *British Journal of Nursing*, **5** (2), 105–109.

Panayiotou B.N., Harper G.D., Fotherby M.D., *et al.* (1993) Interarm blood pressure difference in acute hemiplegia. *Journal of the American Geriatric Society*, **41**, 422–423.

PROGRESS Collaborative Group (2001) Randomized trial of a perindopril-based blood pressure lowering regimen among 6105 individuals with previous stroke or transient ischaemic attack. *Lancet*, **358**, 1033–1041.

Royal College of Nursing (2002) *RCN Code of Practice for Patient Handling*, 2nd edn. London, Royal College of Nursing.

Royal College of Physicians (2000) *National Clinical Guidelines for Stroke*. Suffolk, Lavenham Press.

Royal College of Physicians (2004) *National Clinical Guidelines for Stroke*, 2nd edn. Suffolk, Lavenham Press.

Rud A., Irwin P. and Penhale B. (2000) *Stroke at your fingertips*. London, Class Publishing.

The Stroke Unit Trialists' Collaboration (1997) Collaborative systematic review of the randomized trials of organised inpatient (stroke unit) care after stroke. *British Medical Journal*, **314**, 1151–1159.

The Stroke Unit Trialists' Collaboration (2001) Organised inpatient (stroke unit) care for stroke. *The Cochrane Database of Systematic Reviews*, Issue 3. Art No.: CD000197. DOI: 10.1002/14651858. CD000197. http://www.cochrane.org/

Von Kummer R., Allen K.L., Holle R., *et al.* (1997) Acute stroke: usefulness of early CT findings before thrombolytic therapy. *Radiology*, **205**, 327–333.

Wardlaw J., del Zoppo G., Yamaguchi T. and Berge E. (2004) Thrombolysis for acute ishaemic stroke. *The Cochrane Database of Systematic Reviews*, Issue 3. Art No.: CD00213. DOI: 10.1002/14651858. CD000213. http://www.cochrane.org/

Warlow C.P., Dennis M.S., van Gijn J., *et al.* (2001) *Stroke. A Practical Guide to Management*. Oxford, Blackwell Science.

Williams B., Poulter N., Brown M., *et al.* (2004) Guidelines for management of hypertension: report of the fourth working party of the British Hypertension Society 2004 – BHS IV. *Journal of Human Hypertension*, **18**, 139–185.

Wolfe C., Rudd A. and Beech R. (1996) *Stroke Services and Research. An Overview with Recommendations for Future Research*. London, The Stroke Association.

Wolfe C., Rudd A., Howard R., Coshall C., *et al.* (2002) Incidence and case fatality rates of stroke subtypes in a multiethnic population: the South London stroke register. *Journal of Neurology, Neurosurgery and Psychiatry*, **72**, 211–216.

World Health Organization (1978) *Cerebrovascular Disorders: A Clinical and Research Classification*. Geneva, WHO, Offset Publication No. 43.

World Health Organization (1980) *International Classification of Impairments, Disabilities and Handicaps. Conference Papers*. Geneva, WHO.

World Health Organization (2001) *International Classification of Functioning, Disability and Health: ICF*. Geneva, WHO.

Chapter 9
Rehabilitation of Patients with an Acquired Brain Injury or a Degenerative Neuromuscular Disorder

Debbie Peniket and Rosie Grove

Introduction

Nursing practice has been described as both an art and a science and is informed by a body of knowledge drawn from many different disciplines. In most fields of nursing practice one paradigm can be said to dominate. For example, in the operating theatre or intensive care unit, if the patient is to survive the rigors of surgery the dominant paradigm must be science. Rehabilitation of any kind requires a broad knowledge base because it has holism as a core concept. In neurorehabilitation this multi-paradigmatic approach is essential because the nervous system not only regulates our physiology but also our way of perceiving and interpreting the world around us. The person who has suffered damage to this system may have innumerable and complex problems. To practise effectively in neurorehabilitation an advanced knowledge of human physiology and pathophysiology is essential, but is not enough in isolation. Wider issues about what it means to be a person and how a person constructs and reconstructs his personal reality and identity need to be understood and addressed. The context in which the illness occurs also needs to be considered. In short, neurorehabilitation is one of the most challenging and rewarding fields of endeavour for advanced practice in nursing.

This chapter considers the challenges and opportunities facing those working as advanced practitioners in the field of neurorehabilitation. General principles are illustrated and illuminated by case studies. A focus on the management of two common neurological conditions provides insight into universal neurological problems, and demonstrates the breadth and diversity of this field of practice. Indicative content includes:

- Definition of neurorehabilitation
- Epidemiology: the challenge of numbers
- The challenge of stigma

- The opportunity for education
- The challenge of enduring disability
- The opportunity for integrated team working
- The challenge of assessment
- The opportunity for professional development
- The challenge and opportunity of service development
- Advanced practice in traumatic brain injury
- Advanced practice in multiple sclerosis

Definition of neurorehabilitation

Rehabilitation in this context goes beyond the time-limited, intervention-focused discipline, developed to improve function and favoured by the proponents of intermediate care. Neurorehabilitation can be an ongoing process carried out over the course of the person's lifespan, and delivered in a variety of settings. It is a person-centred process with a broad-spectrum approach that facilitates and enhances quality of life. Neurorehabilitation has been defined as, 'an active and dynamic process by which a disabled person is helped to acquire knowledge and skills in order to maximise physical, psychological and social function.' (Barnes & Radermacher, 2003). There are three main approaches: to reduce impairment; to promote adaptation through the acquisition of new skills or strategies; and to reduce disability by working to remove social and physical barriers in the environment that inhibit participation.

Epidemiology: the challenge of numbers

Neurological conditions are common. Indeed they are the most common cause of serious disability in the Western world, having a significant impact on health and social care services and accounting for 19% of all hospital admissions. It has been estimated that 10 million people in the UK are living with a neurological condition that has a significant impact on their lives (Neurological Alliance, 2003). The prevalence of these chronic conditions is rising due to a combination of increased longevity and improved diagnostic techniques and treatment. There is also an increased prevalence of neurological conditions in older people as some conditions particularly affect older people. These figures are predicted to rise sharply in the next two decades and have been identified as a major challenge to service delivery both in the UK and internationally (World Health Organization, 2002). The impact of these figures on individuals and on health and care delivery can be illustrated by the following statistics provided by the Neurological Alliance:

- Over 1 million people in the UK (2% of the population) are disabled by their neurological condition.
- 350 000 people require help for most of their daily living activities.

- Each year 600 000 people are newly diagnosed with a neurological condition.
- 10% of visits to accident and emergency (A&E) departments are for a neurological problem.
- 17% of GP consultations are for neurological symptoms.
- 30% of people attending A&E departments for head injury are children of 15 years and under.
- 25% of people aged between 16 and 64 years of age with chronic disability have a neurological condition.
- Approximately one-third of disabled people living in residential care have a neurological condition.
- Approximately 850 000 people in the UK care for someone with a neurological condition.

Further statistics demonstrating the magnitude of both the incidence and prevalence of key neurological conditions is provided in Table 9.1.

Table 9.1 Incidence and prevalence of key neurological conditions (Neurological Alliance, 2003).

Condition	Incidence (number of new cases that develop each year in brackets)	Prevalence: total number of people per 100 000 (number with the condition in the UK in brackets)
Brain injury	Severe injury 10–15 Moderate injury 15–20 Mild injury 250–300	228 with long-term problems (135 000)
Brain tumour	20 per 100 000 (12 000)	
Cerebral palsy		186 (110 000)
Epilepsy	89 per 100 000	500 (300 000)
Guillain–Barré syndrome	2.5 per 100 000 (1500)	
Motor neurone disease	2 per 100 000	7 per 100 000 (4000 approx.)
Multiple sclerosis	4 per 100 000 (2500)	144 (85 000)
Parkinson's disease	17 per 100 000 (10 000 approx.)	200 (120 000)
Stroke	240 per 100 000 (100 000)	500 (300 000)

Challenges and opportunities for advanced/specialist nursing roles in neurorehabilitation

Challenge: stigma

Despite the large numbers of individuals affected, members of the general public often have little insight into the consequences of a neurological condition until they have direct personal experience. Levels of awareness are low even about relatively common conditions such as epilepsy and head injury. Conditions that are less common, such as Friedreich's ataxia, are largely unheard of and poorly understood by both the general public and health and social care professionals alike. Research commissioned to underpin the National Service Framework (NSF) for Long-term Conditions demonstrates the fear felt by patients who perceive that the professionals organising and delivering their care have little understanding of their particular needs (Hardy, 2002). Individuals with conditions affecting their ability to communicate are particularly vulnerable and often disadvantaged by the failure of staff to recognise the extent to which this problem affects care. Similarly, busy staff may wrongly interpret cognitive and behavioural problems and attribute any difficulties to personality defects, failure to adjust or obstinacy. These labels once acquired are often difficult to shake off, becoming accepted and perpetuated by other health professionals without further investigation or assessment. In this way the ignorance and attitudes of others can compound the difficulties people with neurological conditions experience, often causing them to feel stigmatised and misunderstood, which can, in turn, lead to further social, emotional and economic disadvantage.

Opportunity: education

Rehabilitation is an education-based discipline and it is imperative that staff and patients understand the process and purpose of their labours so they can work together to achieve the best possible outcome. An important part of the advanced/specialist practitioner role is to provide education and information while modelling best evidence-based practice. A specialist nurse in neurological rehabilitation may be required to visit patients in many different settings, for example in an intensive care unit or community hospital, nursing home or the patient's own home. Whatever the venue the object is always to support the rehabilitation process by working in partnership with patients and care providers. Sometimes the nurse will be required to be a patient advocate, spending time modelling the process of early assessment, establishing motivating factors and identifying appropriate patient-centred goals. Another occasion may provide the opportunity to share and explore concerns, provide information or perhaps advise on a more formal training opportunity. The advanced practitioner in rehabilitation needs to use the same nurturing practices to encourage growth and learning in his/her colleagues as he/she does with patients and their families. The following example illustrates the benefit of this approach to both the individual patient and the wider health care community as a whole.

Case study

Peter was a 28-year-old man who had suffered profound anoxic brain damage as a result of a road traffic accident. He had been placed in a local community hospital where he was to continue his rehabilitation until adaptations could be completed on his property.

Peter was able to see and respond to his surroundings and the people around him, but he was unable to communicate consistently and therefore formal assessment of his perception and cognition had been limited. He had some voluntary movement of all four limbs but no sitting balance, and was considered to be profoundly dyspraxic. He also had high tone with frequent extensor spasms and clonus. When staff tried to wash and dress Peter they faced great difficulty wrestling with rigid arms and legs, and no matter how much they remonstrated with him, or tried to distract him, he would cry out continually and fight against them. There appeared to be no reason for his actions. This behaviour came to be viewed by them as deliberately obstructive and his care would be rushed because of the distress his behaviour caused to the staff. By the time the morning routine had been completed Peter was too upset and tired to eat and would spend miserable mornings unable to maintain a good position in his chair. The nurses and therapists felt very sorry for Peter, but also profoundly frustrated because they could not engage him in activities and they believed there was nothing they could do to improve his quality of life. The team's relationship with Peter's mother also became strained and the team began to avoid her and dread caring for him.

Intervention
The specialist nurse in rehabilitation was able to discuss these issues with the multidisciplinary team and, in partnership with them, undertook a review of Peter's physical impairments exploring the assumptions behind the team's interventions. Discussing the nature of his impairments enabled the nursing team to realise that although Peter could 'see', his perception was severely hampered by his loss of tactile/kinaesthetic sensation and his difficulty interpreting information. Their attempts at distraction were actually making the situation worse by overloading his already overstretched powers of perception and compromising his ability to interpret information successfully: the equivalent of encouraging a learner driver to engage in conversation, play music loudly and negotiate a busy roundabout while sending a text message!

The specialist nurse was also able to lead a multidisciplinary reflective practice session, encouraging the staff to consider the effect Peter's actions had on their behaviour. This meeting enabled the team to explore their core beliefs about rehabilitation, and allowed them to examine why they were feeling and reacting as they were and what were their own learning needs in this situation.

The consequences for the team
As a result of this cathartic discussion, the specialist nurse arranged with the ward manager that a neurophysiotherapist, who worked exclusively with individuals who have severe head injuries, to work with the team both as a group and on a one-to-one basis with Peter and his mother to demonstrate the best way to approach his daily care. A video was made of his morning routine to use as a teaching aid for new staff. When Peter was discharged the video was also employed as part of the induction package for his new

carers. The ward team were keen to pass on their new learning to both the carers and his family thus improving the quality of the relationship between the staff and Peter's mother.

The consequences for Peter

Peter was able to participate in many of the morning activities and his rigidity decreased. Although he was still noisy on occasions, the quality of his interaction with the staff improved considerably. Following his morning routine, a short period of relaxing, positioned rest enabled him to sit more comfortably in his chair and engage in other social interaction. When he was discharged from hospital the continuity of approach was maintained by the use of the training video.

This mixed approach, of providing specialist knowledge while exploring and challenging underlying beliefs, enables development and growth in colleagues and models the principles of good rehabilitative practice. It creates greater confidence in practitioners, providing them with insight that leads to better relationships with patients and their relatives. This, in turn, has benefits not only for one patient but also for all future patients that pass through that environment.

Challenge: enduring disability

Neurological conditions are many and varied in their presentation and course. Some illnesses are degenerative over time, for example motor neurone disease; others are subject to relapse and remission (e.g., multiple sclerosis), while still others are amenable to either treatment (e.g., myasthenia gravis), or cure (e.g., meningitis). The onset may be insidious or catastrophic: the course may be unpredictable or relentlessly progressive. These factors make it extremely difficult to anticipate and plan for both the day-to-day management and the future.

As many of the conditions become apparent or occur in young adulthood, the impact of this sudden change in fortune and difficulty in planning for the future goes beyond the individual directly affected. It can have a significant impact on the individual's family. Therefore, planning appropriate packages of care requires an assessment not only of individual need but also of the needs of the family. However, no situation remains static over time and the family, like the individual and indeed the disease process, is dynamic and evolving.

Case study

A 40-year-old man with transverse myelitis was discharged to live at home with his wife and two children. At the time of his discharge the children were 12 and 10 years of age. Adaptations made to the family home enabled John to be carried from the bedroom to the bathroom by an overhead hoist. Over the door to the family bathroom, there was a large gap that enabled the overhead hoist and tracking to pass over the landing and into John's bedroom directly opposite. This fixture prevented any member of the family from using the bathroom with privacy. As the family grew up this became a huge issue and a strain on the relationships, which eventually led to a prolonged period of hospitalisation and review, in order to re-evaluate the situation and provide more suitable housing.

It is of course difficult to judge how much the poor adaptations played a part in the strains that developed, but John's wife, Mary, explained how the situation evolved with the following story. When the second child, Julie, began her periods, Mary set about reassuring her and talked her through ways of coping. She asked Julie whether she had any preference for a particular type of sanitary goods. She replied that she didn't mind as long as there was no rustling wrapping paper to take off because she didn't want her father or his carers to hear her when she was in the bathroom. The adaptation of a small family bathroom for one person's use may have had little impact when the children were young, but no thought had been given to the family's developing needs. While this problem was acknowledged by community staff as it developed, no action was taken until the situation had broken down.

It is vital, therefore, for the advanced practitioner to be accessible, flexible and responsive enough to manage these changes. Without proactive management, review and re-assessment, the individual's home situation may become untenable or the client may develop secondary complications such as pressure sores or contractures that are as much, if not more, disabling than the presenting condition. Over time, this model of practice can result in the development of close working relationships with the individual and their families. This relationship can be rewarding, but the challenge for the practitioner is to manage the potential dependency that may develop over time by promoting personal autonomy and maintaining therapeutic boundaries.

Opportunity: integrated team working

This chapter will not attempt to define the roles and responsibilities of the rehabilitation team, but will identify the benefits of team working in relation to the management of neurological conditions and the support that team members can offer each other. However, it must be acknowledged that the word 'team' can mean different things to different people. For example, the British Society for Rehabilitation Medicine (BSRM) conducted a survey of community rehabilitation teams and received responses from single practitioners working with a virtual team of colleagues from other disciplines, as well as the traditional established model of multidisciplinary team. Whilst there are distinct advantages to working within an established team that share a base, this is not essential to effective team working. It may be that an individual working with a virtual team (i.e. a geographically disparate group of professionals who function as a team by making use of communication technology) could draw together a broader expertise from different agencies. This can generate creative thinking and equally valid 'team work'. Evidence suggests that a team approach, as a way of working, is also very acceptable to clients (Oxtoby, 1999).

The key benefits identified include:

- Continuity of care: a team offers continuity of contact, which can avoid duplication of assessment and information. Symptoms experienced by people with long-term neurological conditions can be difficult to describe and there are clear advantages in meeting with team members who are familiar with the situation. The key worker or case manager role provides this continuity in a virtual team and can also ensure the best use of scarce resources.
- Development of professional expertise: as some of the neurological conditions mentioned are relatively rare and variable in their signs and symptoms, it is difficult for general practitioners, general nurses and therapists to build up specialist knowledge and expertise. The team approach allows for the development of such expertise and can offer a resource for other professionals working in different settings. The advanced practitioner can make a significant contribution to this cross-fertilisation of knowledge and is ideally placed to undertake the key worker/care manager role.
- Increased support for both the client and team worker: by the provision of support and information that acknowledges and addresses the emotional, practical and social aspects of the individual's situation, the team can assist in preventing the feelings of helplessness that can often accompany long-term illness.

Case study

In April 2001, John was diagnosed with Guillain–Barré syndrome (GBS), an acute inflammatory disease of the nervous system causing polyneuropathy. He spent eight months in an acute hospital trust before being transferred to the inpatient neurorehabilitation unit (INRU) situated within the local community hospital, in December 2001. He had spent four of the eight months in the intensive care unit where he received ventilatory support. John and his partner were visited by the nurse consultant whilst still in the acute setting in order to:

- Discuss and plan his transfer
- Give John and his partner information on the unit
- Discuss his progress and current rehabilitation programme with the team involved in his care
- Support identification of his goals and priorities
- Identify any issues that the team on the INRU needed to be aware of in preparation for his transfer

- Begin to develop the relationship with John and his family that would be called upon as he faced the long and difficult journey ahead.

This early identification of goals proved extremely helpful to the team. Upon meeting with John for the first time, it was apparent that his mood was very low and he held little optimism for the future. The one wish he did express was to be with his family on Christmas day. As John had barely been out of bed let alone out on a home visit, this presented quite a challenge. Together, the team in the acute trust and the team from the INRU worked on a plan that would give John the best possible chance to achieve this goal. We believed that this would offer him a major psychological boost that would ultimately impact positively on his rehabilitation.

John was transferred to the unit on the 13th December and the team really did pull out all the stops. On Christmas day he spent three hours with his family at home with no ill effects. It was a tremendous achievement for him (and the team) and it really did lift his spirits and, in turn, his hopes for the future.

John continued to set challenging goals. One very unusual request was to marry his long-term partner in the hospital's chapel. With a special licence from the Archbishop of Canterbury, a very supportive hospital chaplain, a fellow patient as best man and a lot of willing volunteers, another of John's 'goals' was achieved. He did indeed marry his partner in the hospital chapel on February 14th 2002.

It is important to recognise that this 'emotional labour' (Smith, 1992) can also have an impact upon team members. Working with people who have incurable, progressive conditions can be rewarding but also very demanding. The team approach enables members to derive support from each other, and are therefore more able to cope with the inevitable stresses encountered in continuing to meet the patients' and families' needs.

The following example demonstrates how one team led by a specialist health visitor in physical disability, identified this need and initiated a model of clinical supervision to strengthen the support within the team and to enhance clinical and professional practice.

Wyre Forest Community Rehabilitation Team (formerly the disability team) was established in 1991 to support the needs of individuals aged 16–64 years with physical disabilities. The team comprised a specialist health visitor in physical disability, specialist nurses in brain injury and neurology, an occupational therapist, physiotherapist and speech and language therapist. The caseload was varied and included individuals with spinal injury, brain injury and a variety of neurodegenerative and neuromuscular conditions. The team aimed to support individuals to live independently within the community, to make informed choices with regard to their treatment and care and to realise their aspirations wherever possible. The impact of working with younger people with these often very debilitating diseases became evident when case discussions were held within team meetings. It was therefore agreed to undertake clinical supervision as a team in order to address the challenging and often emotional aspects of the work.

Over a decade ago, the Department of Health (DH) published *A Vision for the Future: The Nursing, Midwifery and Health Visiting Contribution to Health and Healthcare* (DH, 1993). Clinical supervision was then defined as: 'a formal process of professional support and learning which enables individual practitioners to develop knowledge and competence, assume responsibility for their own practice and enhance consumer protection and safety in complex situations' (DH, 1993). The idea of clinical supervision as defined above only developed during the late 1980s and early 1990s, having been generally accepted as standard practice in social work and psychotherapy.

The Community Rehabilitation Team (CRT) felt that this framework had many benefits to offer, not only the supportive aspects but also the opportunity to develop knowledge and professional practice. After the CRT had agreed a model of group supervision and the ground rules that were to be used, the specialist health visitor sought an appropriate facilitator from a clinical psychology background, who would support the process and provide insight into the group's experience. The CRT allocated one hour per month for group clinical supervision, in addition to some time for preparation and follow-up if required. The benefits were quickly felt by all team members and it soon became an integral part of practice. Team members identified some of the positive aspects, as follows:

- Lessened feelings of isolation
- Improved confidence and competence
- Offered the opportunity to reflect on clinical decision-making
- Allowed the team to share ideas
- Team members felt more supported
- Team members felt safe to explore the emotional aspects of their role

Several years on and with some changes to the team membership, clinical supervision remains a valuable aspect of the team's activities.

Challenge: assessment

The challenge of assessment is not within the procedure itself but is within the processes required to understand, interpret and apply the information presented. It may be impossible to interview or obtain an accurate history from an individual who has impaired perception or communication, resulting in confusion and gaps in understanding of the situation. An even more confused and distorted picture may be obtained from the patient with cognitive impairment whose lack of insight and memory loss may bring about the construction of an entirely false history. An advanced practitioner will be aware of these problems and will apply theoretical knowledge and interpersonal skills in order to make detailed observation and provide skilful prompts that inform the process of history construction and assessment.

It is then possible to construct a rehabilitation programme that takes account of both the macro and the micro picture, i.e. the individual's whole circumstances and the subtlest impairment. In any rehabilitation process there is a need for careful observation and application of theoretical knowledge, but in neurorehabilitation the entire process may be jeopardised if there is a failure to interpret the information and observation skilfully. For example, a previously articulate and well-read businessman finding himself unable to read following a cerebral bleed, disguised this problem by appearing to read the newspaper. If this had not been identified following discharge, the ongoing rehabilitation programme would have been severely compromised by the lack of information that he could access and the failure to involve a speech and language therapist.

Opportunity: professional development

Neurorehabilitation offers the opportunity to work closely with specialists in other disciplines, including neurologists, orthopaedic surgeons, urologists and gastroenterologists, psychologists and counsellors, to name but a few. This provides an endless resource for all rehabilitation nurses wishing to advance their skills and practice. There are also more formal avenues for professional development in the form of post-registration education pathways and advanced health assessment programmes. This is an exciting time for nurses to embark upon new initiatives. Indeed, the strategic importance of the nurses' role in the NHS was underlined in *Making a Difference* (DH, 1999) and subsequently enlarged upon in *Liberating the Talents* and *The Ten Key Roles for Nurses* (DH, 2002) This presents opportunities to develop innovative nurse-led services.

Service delivery: a challenge and an opportunity

Traditionally, the provision of services for these patients grew up around individual practitioners' interests and specialties. Surveys regarding the number and function of community-based neurorehabilitation teams were undertaken to inform the BSRM in the development of standards for community-based rehabilitation. These indicate that provision is patchy and extremely variable in the quality and quantity of the interventions offered (McMillan & Ledder, 2001; Turner-Stokes, *et al.*, 2001). This state of affairs offers both a challenge and an opportunity, as it offers the possibility of redesigning or delivering new services to meet the needs of those currently not being addressed.

The announcement in February 2001 regarding the development of a National Service Framework (NSF) for Long-term Conditions offers a real opportunity to focus on the needs of people with neurological disorders, and to consider some of the generic issues of relevance to a wide range of people with long-term conditions and disabilities. This NSF is a 'blueprint' for care, aimed at raising standards, reducing this variation in services, improving the patient experience, increasing compliance with evidence-based practice and providing services to people more quickly. It consists of user-focused quality requirements, representing a set of aims and outcomes that services should aspire to meet. The NSF has been developed in the context of a more devolved NHS; rather than setting national targets and milestones, this NSF provides a 'blueprint' for the Health Care Commission and the Commission for Social Care and Inspection to use as a benchmark for measuring progress. Service users will have an opportunity to influence service delivery and to measure progress through the patient and public forum.

Chronic disease management offers a further opportunity and is on the public health agenda both internationally (WHO, 2002) and nationally (DH, 2004). Successful chronic disease management requires a paradigm shift from reactive medicine to proactive health promotion. This requires health and social professionals to engage in a reappraisal of the prevailing systems of service delivery, and to develop protocols that will enable the implementation of guidelines for best practice and develop pathways to manage the care episode. The course of some neurological conditions runs across the lifespan and may require a transition from child, education-based services to adult-based services. This presents a challenge to the continuity of service provision and offers a real opportunity to integrate services across these artificial organisational barriers. The NSF and the Chronic Disease Management Agenda are both reliant on the successful integration of health and social care, presenting further opportunities for joined-up working.

The integration of social services and health provides an opportunity to develop services for those who have needs that do not fall neatly into existing models of service provision. People with traumatic brain injuries, for example, may have no physical disability, no mental illness, no language or sensory impairment and yet be unable to live at home without daily support and supervision. Assessment of these hidden disabilities and planning effective rehabilitation for these individuals is precisely the sort of area in which an advanced practitioner can make a difference.

Advanced practice in traumatic brain injury

Traumatic Brain Injury (TBI), like stroke, is common and can be extremely complex. When combined together, TBI and stroke make up the largest proportion of cases of acquired brain injury in the United Kingdom (British Society of Rehabilitation Medicine & Royal College of Physicians, 2003). Stroke rehabilitation has received a great deal of attention over the last decade and has now become a major focus of research and resources. Indeed, there is a whole chapter in this book dedicated to the subject. However, although both stroke and TBI can be classified together as acquired brain injury, there are essential differences in the two conditions that make them worthy of separate consideration:

- Stroke tends to occur predominantly in the older population; TBI in the younger age group, with a large number of children and young people affected.
- Over half of all those presenting with a head injury are children under the age of 16 years. It has been suggested that the concentration of TBI in younger people may be an advantage, in that the younger brain has more capacity to recover (cerebral plasticity) (Miller *et al.*, 1990). However, the consequences of a head injury during childhood or adolescence can impact upon education, social skills acquisition and peer relationships often resulting in a lifelong struggle with disability and dependence.
- Stroke occurs more commonly in females, TBI in males.
- Stroke is more common in people with certain predisposing medical conditions; TBI is more commonly associated with those who have certain psychosocial characteristics, such as risk-taking behaviour or substance abuse.
- Although both conditions cause brain damage, they are different in the mechanism and consequences of the injury. Stroke occurs as a result of an internal focal event. TBI is caused by external mechanical forces, and often results in diffuse damage to the brain rather than damage to a particular localised region. Even when there is a clear focal lesion there is usually widespread disruption or stretching of the nerve fibres in the cerebral hemispheres. Consequently, a broad spectrum of cognitive dysfunction may be found following even a 'mild' head injury.

These differences in the natural history of the condition are mirrored by a corresponding disparity in people's understanding and provision for their needs. The individual who has sustained a stroke is likely to have access to a stroke unit or a specialist team of practitioners (in hospital or the community) who have advanced knowledge of the condition and can appreciate and help the individual overcome problems. An individual with TBI is likely to experience a more poorly defined care pathway (Pickard *et al.*, 2004) and consequently may not have access to knowledgeable clinicians. Those who have sustained a mild head injury are frequently not admitted to hospital or referred on to appropriate services, while those with moderate injuries may be admitted to a general orthopaedic ward and discharged with a 'head injury' leaflet. Subsequent problems are often hidden from the general view and consequently underestimated or misunderstood, despite their persistent and significant impact on the individual and their family (Thornhill *et al.*, 2000).

To try to promote a more consistent and effective approach a considerable number of guidance documents on this condition and its management has been produced and this information is summarised in Table 9.2. This field of

Table 9.2 Summary of guidance available for traumatic brain injury and its management.

Document	Date	Organisation
Rehabilitation after traumatic brain injury	1998	British Society of Rehabilitation Medicine (BSRM)
Management of patients with head injuries	1999	Royal College of Surgeons
Health Select Committee: Inquiry into head injury rehabilitation	2001	Department of Health
Guidelines for head injury (first 48 hours)	2003	NICE
Rehabilitation following acquired brain injury. National clinical guidelines	2003	BSRM and RCP Guidelines

neurorehabilitation is therefore fertile ground to be cultivated through education and service development by the advanced practitioner.

Epidemiology: a 'silent epidemic'

The number of individuals affected by TBI is growing. It has a wide range of causes: occurring as a result of road traffic accidents (RTAs), domestic violence or assaults, sports injuries or simple falls. Approximately a million people a year in the United Kingdom sustain a head injury severe enough to warrant a visit to A&E. However, only 10% of these are classified as moderate or severe injuries (Kay & Teasdale, 2001). RTAs cause most of the cases of severe traumatic brain injury, and are likely to become the third most common cause of death and disability worldwide by 2020 (Murray & Lopez, 1997). However, the severity of the injuries sustained does not always correlate with the extent of the residual disability experienced by the individual in the community. Indeed, even those people who sustain 'mild head injuries' may suffer major consequences, such as loss of social interaction, diminished vocational expertise and erosion of close family relationships (Thornhill *et al.*, 2000).

TBI has been included in this chapter because it is a condition that often challenges traditional health care settings and is frequently misunderstood by staff with no specialist knowledge of the condition. It has been estimated that 90% of individuals with severe head injuries make a good physical recovery (Powell, 1994). This lack of visible physical disability contributes to the underestimation of the impact of the injury on an individual's day-to-day life.

Case study

Tom, a middle-aged man, was discharged from hospital following a short stay in an orthopaedic ward as a result of sustaining a mild head injury at work. Tom's only problems appeared to be a tendency to muddle his words and difficulty remembering new information. His family were told that this would improve gradually, he was referred to the speech therapist and they were given no special instructions on discharge. Three weeks later the speech therapist visited Tom's home at the request of his wife and found the situation near to breaking point. His wife and daughter had discovered it was unsafe to leave Tom alone. In the first few days after discharge he had put all the clean washing stacked and ready for ironing in black bags and left them out for the dustmen, vacuumed up the artificial coals in their 'Living Flame' fire and flooded the bathroom having left the taps running for a bath and then forgotten all about it. To add to the tension, Tom did not believe there was a problem and became extremely angry and non-cooperative when supervised. Tom was referred to a community specialist Acquired Brain Injury (ABI) team and made considerable progress. However, despite their best efforts he was unable to return to work.

This case study illustrates how an individual may be profoundly disabled by traumatic brain damage and yet appears (and believes himself to be) perfectly able.

Pathology and classification of traumatic brain injury

A head injury may be referred to according to the direct impact of the trauma as a 'closed' or 'penetrating' injury. A penetrating injury occurs as a result of an object penetrating the scalp, fracturing the skull and piercing the brain. This is less common than a closed head injury, in which an external force creates a violent movement within the brain that damages the structures within it.

An RTA, for example, results in rapid acceleration, deceleration and sometimes also rotation of the brain within the skull. As a result of these sudden movements there is a widespread disruption of the neuronal pathways, and sometimes blood vessels acting like cheese wires cut through the softer neuronal structures. In an older person the blood vessels may be more friable and frequently bleed. Damage is also incurred to the frontal and temporal lobes of the brain as the soft brain tissue is moved over the surface of the bony prominences inside the skull. The frontal lobes are responsible for higher intellectual functions such as planning and organisation, as well as the control of behaviour and emotions. It is also the seat of personality, with a small area called the 'anterior cingulated cortex' believed to contain the 'I' we all feel we have inside us. The temporal lobes are concerned with memory (both long-term memories and procedural memories are stored there) and language. Depending upon the force of the impact, reciprocal damage to the occipital lobe (concerned with vision) may occur as the brain rebounds from the front of the skull to the back.

Secondary to the damage sustained at the point of trauma, there may also be damage caused by anoxia or subsequent pathological processes such as swelling and haemorrhage. The most consistent effect of diffuse brain disorder is loss of consciousness caused by the disruption of connections between the reticular formation and the cortex. This may be very transient (a matter of moments), or last for days, weeks or months.

Table 9.3 Classification of head injury (Rosenthal *et al.*, 1990).

• **Minor:**	GCS > 15
• **Mild:**	GCS 13–15, LOC < 20 mins, PTA < 24 h
• **Moderate:**	GCS 9–12, LOC 20 min–36 h, PTA 1–7 days
• **Severe:**	GCS 3–8, LOC > 36 h, PTA > 7 days

Abbreviations: GCS, Glasgow Coma Scale; LOC, loss of consciousness; PTA, post-traumatic amnesia.

Table 9.4 Potential deficits arising from acquired brain injury. Reproduced from BSRM (2003).

Physical	Communicative	Cognitive	Behavioural/emotional
Motor deficits: Paralysis, abnormal muscle tone, ataxia/ poor coordination	*Language deficits:* Expression Comprehension Dysarthria Dyslexia Dysgraphia	*Impairment of:* Memory Attention Perception Problem-solving Insight	Emotional lability Poor initiation Mood change Adjustment problems Aggressive outbursts Disinhibition
Sensory deficits: Visual/olfactory/ hearing loss *Symptoms:* Headache, fatigue, pain, dysphagia, seizures		Safety Self-monitoring Social judgement	Inappropriate sexual behaviour Poor motivation Psychosis

Classification of the severity of a head injury is based on three main indicators:

- The severity of the injury on admission as measured by the score on the Glasgow Coma Scale (GCS).
- The length of time the individual experiences loss of consciousness (LOC).
- The period (often following coma) during which the patient appears to be awake and aware but is still cerebrally disordered: often described as being in a 'waking dream' because the patient has no memory of events – known as post-traumatic amnesia (PTA).

Table 9.3 provides a summary of the classification of head injury.

Potential problems encountered following TBI

Traumatic brain injury, like stroke, can present as a mixed picture of deficits, as Table 9.4 illustrates, with each person being affected in a particular, individual manner. Many of these deficits will be manifest with a tangible, measurable effect. However, some losses are only made apparent in the qualities of the individual's interactions. The person is quite literally 'not himself'. In order to establish if this has happened or the extent of the change that has taken place, it is vital to take a good history from the person's family. Relatives report that the ten most difficult problems to deal with are:

- Personality change
- Slowness
- Poor memory
- Irritability
- Bad temper
- Depression
- Tiredness
- Rapid mood changes
- Tension and anxiety
- Threats of violence

In some individuals these problems may only be evident in the early days during the period of post-traumatic amnesia, but for others the problems will persist throughout their lives. The advanced practitioner can have a positive impact in either setting: in the early days in hospital or by negotiating appropriate care and support in the community, as the next case study demonstrates.

Post-traumatic amnesia

'Post-traumatic amnesia' (PTA) is a term used to describe the time between injury and the recovery of continuous memory. First used as a measure in the 1930s, it was suggested that the length of time taken to recover consciousness indicates the quantity of brain tissue damaged, and the return of memory for day-to-day events is the last stage in the restoration of full consciousness (Russell, 1932). PTA is a confusional state often characterised by the semblance of normality, such as being able to talk, walk and engage in quite complex tasks, for example using a mobile telephone.
    Manifestations of PTA:

- Poor memory
- Agitation
- Lack of insight
- Disorientation
- Attention disorder
- Anger and irritability
- Disinhibition

The early management of individuals with mild to moderate head injuries tends to take place on busy acute wards and it is rarely viewed as a problem when the patients are in a drowsy, immobile state. However, as the patient progresses from unconsciousness to PTA and becomes confused and disruptive, this can create considerable problems for both the individual with brain

injury and the other patients and staff on the ward. An inappropriate environment quickly generates physical and behavioural complications, and these
problems can be exacerbated by the use of sedative medications to control
the patient's agitation (Fleminger, 2003). This has an adverse effect on the
patient's progress, with recent research indicating a direct correlation between
the length of time a person spends in an acute environment following the
stabilisation of their medical condition and the number of bed days required
for inpatient rehabilitation (Sirois *et al.*, 2004). As the NICE guidelines state:
'Once patients are medically and surgically stable, their continued stay in an
acute unit is clinically counterproductive and the simple act of transfer to the
calmer, quieter atmosphere of a rehabilitation unit has benefits on cognition
and outcome.'

The advanced practitioner's role in these circumstances is to not only over-
see the management of signs and symptoms so as to reduce complications, but
also to negotiate and promote rehabilitation pathways appropriate to the individual's needs.

Case study

Robert, a 35-year-old man, sustained a blow to his head as a result of a
heavy fall while intoxicated. He was admitted to an orthopaedic ward for
observation. As his conscious level lifted he became more vocal as well as
more active, walking about the ward in a very unsteady way using any
furniture to hand to maintain his balance. He repeatedly walked up to the
nurses' station and banged on the desk, and frequently walked into the female
area of the ward where he would either behave in a sexually inappropriate
manner or pass urine or open his bowels in the corner. He was irritable and
physically obdurate when challenged.

Robert was known to some of the ward team who lived locally. They
reported that he drank heavily and normally behaved in an unrestrained,
threatening manner. The nurse consultant was called for in the light of his
behaviour and asked to review Robert, with the intention of moving him to
a secure unit where he would not be putting himself or others at risk.

Nurse consultant interventions

Assessment: A thorough holistic assessment is vital to fully understand the
situation and develop an effective plan. This includes an educational and
vocational history, as well as information about the family and home
environment. Reading carefully through his extensive notes and engaging
his family in conversation revealed an interesting pre-morbid history. Robert
had dropped out of school at 15 and worked as a delivery boy for a local
butcher. He was a cheerful boy who was very keen on fishing and had won
many cups in competitions. He was admitted to hospital overnight aged 16
following an accident on his pushbike that had rendered him unconscious

for a short period. Over the next 19 years Robert's character changed. He lost all interest in activities, was admitted fifteen times with head injuries caused by assaults, falls and road traffic accidents. He had treatment for alcohol dependency, suffered depression and made two attempts at suicide. He had not been in regular work since his first accident and his family had, in despair, largely disowned him.

The consequences

In collaboration with the multidisciplinary team the nurse consultant reviewed his current physiological state. Robert was being prescribed a regular dose of haloperidol to control his agitation. This was replaced with carbamazepine to mediate his mood. Gradually, as he became less drowsy, his speech became more intelligible and it became apparent that he was disorientated in time and place. He thought that the nurses' station was a bar and was banging on the surface to attract the 'barmaid's' attention.

In order to reduce the distractions and irritations in his environment it was agreed to move Robert into a single room. However, to ensure appropriate observation and supervision, the nurse consultant negotiated with the hospital management team for an extra member of staff to observe, monitor and record his behaviour.

The multidisciplinary team collaborated in developing proactive strategies to manage some of his undesirable behaviour. For example, encouraging him to use the lavatory regularly reduced the instances of incontinence. The desire to wander was controlled by creating a safe circuit that avoided turning round but gave the impression of freedom and progress. These strategies were recorded in his care plan to ensure continuity and consistency of approach. A more relaxed atmosphere reduced the stress on his parents and lessened the feelings of shame and guilt.

Robert's parents became active partners in the decision-making process regarding his future. He was referred to a rehabilitation consultant and, following discussion, it was decided he would benefit from further therapy at a specialist rehabilitation centre.

Coordination of the transfer process enabled a smooth handover of all the gathered information. This informed and facilitated the speedy development of an effective rehabilitation programme. Identification of a key worker ensured that there would be a similar smooth transition back into his local community.

Consequences for Robert

During the rehabilitation process it became apparent that Robert was severely cognitively impaired and would be unable to live independently. The team believed that this was likely to be the a result of the cumulative damage sustained by his repeated head injuries. However, Robert did not require management in a secure unit as was initially proposed. He now lives in supported housing with other young people who have brain injuries. He no longer drinks alcohol, has a good relationship with his parents and is once more enjoying fishing.

Hippocrates has been attributed with the words, 'No head injury is too trivial to ignore'. Had Robert's first head injury been acknowledged and managed appropriately he may have avoided the self-destructive cycle of behaviour that led to this outcome.

Advanced practice in multiple sclerosis

Multiple sclerosis (MS) is the commonest cause of neurological disability in young adults. It is often diagnosed between the ages of 20 and 45 years, coinciding with key periods and transition points in the family life cycle, thereby impacting on work, career and parenting, amongst others. It follows an uncertain and unpredictable course, and prognosis can vary dramatically from one individual to another. These factors present particular challenges in ensuring that care is responsive, flexible and appropriate to these very individual needs.

Epidemiology of MS

There are few diseases that have such a wealth of information available about their prevalence and incidence worldwide. This information indicates that the prevalence of MS becomes higher with increasing distance from the equator. While MS tends to be rare in countries such as Africa, it is relatively common in Northern Europe, Northern America and Southern Australia. The prevalence around the world varies dramatically from less than 5/100 000 to more than 150/100 000. In the UK there are approximately 85 000 people with MS, the prevalence varying from 115/100 000 in Surrey to 170/100 000 in the Shetlands.

Studies have also shown that the ratio of males to females with MS remains constant at 1:2, as does age of onset. Age of onset of MS tends to be a year or two later in men than in women, but men are more likely to develop severe disease. The average age of onset is 29–33 years. Studies have also shown that the risk of an individual developing MS is multifactorial. While the disease is not hereditary, there is a genetic component thought to make up approximately 25% of an individual's risk factor. The remaining risk is probably due to one or more environmental triggers, which may include diet and climate. The evidence that the immune system plays a central role in the pathogenesis of the disease is overwhelming, whereas the role of infection as a trigger remains unclear but cannot be ruled out.

Pathology and classification of MS

MS affects the central nervous system (CNS), i.e. the brain and spinal cord. To understand the complex processes occurring in MS, it is necessary for the advanced practitioner to have a depth of knowledge in relation to normal anatomy, physiology and immunology.

Pathologically, MS is characterised by areas of focal demyelination (plaques) disseminated throughout the CNS. This has the potential to produce neurological deficits. Given the varied nature and distribution of pathological lesions in MS, it is expected that the disease will present a variety of clinical deficits, or a combination of deficits. Within the many individual variations of MS, some patterns have emerged and five different types of MS have been defined (Burgess, 2002):

- Relapsing–remitting MS
- Secondary progressive MS
- Primary progressive MS
- Benign MS
- Malignant or Marburg's MS

People with MS can experience a wide range of different symptoms. A survey of 656 people with MS (Kraft *et al.*, 1986) listed over 14 different symptoms, each experienced by at least 23% of people. The following is a list of common presenting symptoms:

- Diplopia (double vision)
- Visual deficits (e.g. optic neuritis, nystagmus)
- Poor balance and coordination
- Muscle weakness
- Stiffness or spasticity
- Altered sensation
- Fatigue inappropriate to activity
- Bladder and bowel problems
- Impotence
- Forgetfulness and poor concentration

Burgess (2002) stated that the types of symptoms experienced can be subdivided into primary, secondary and tertiary. Primary symptoms occur as a direct result of demyelination within the CNS, e.g. weakness and bladder dysfunction. Secondary symptoms occur as a result of complications caused by a combination of the primary symptoms and insufficient management of the symptoms, e.g. recurrent urine infections caused by untreated bladder dysfunction. Tertiary symptoms are described as the psychosocial consequences of primary and secondary symptoms, e.g. unemployment, role changes, loss of independence (Holland & Halper, 1999).

Whatever symptoms someone with MS experiences, they can have a major impact on an individual's confidence, self-esteem, role within the family, social life, employment and sexuality.

So when might a person with MS need rehabilitation services? The National Institute for Clinical Excellence (NICE) in their *Clinical Guidelines for the Management of MS in Primary and Secondary Care* (2003), recommend that all people with MS have ready access to a specialist neurological service for:

- Diagnosis of MS initially, and of subsequent symptoms as necessary
- Provision of specific pharmacological treatments especially disease-modifying drugs

The development of the role of specialist nurse in MS, and the competencies identified and published in July 2003, have clearly defined the role and skills required to support an individual with MS in all phases of the disease process. However, people with MS should also have ready access to a specialist neurological rehabilitation service. This should be available when the presenting problem is outside the competence of the first point of contact. The specialist neurological rehabilitation service should provide:

- Assessment when the individual has complex problems
- Specific pharmacological or other therapies
- An integrated programme of rehabilitation
- Monitoring of change
- Advice to other services

Symptom management

This section will not address an exhaustive list of symptoms and their management, rather it will explore how rehabilitation can impact upon two key problems: fatigue and spasticity. These two problems have been chosen as a focus because they epitomise the quantitative and qualitative nature of disease. Spasticity is an observable, measurable phenomenon whereas fatigue is a largely subjective, hidden experience. It has been observed that research into the management and treatment of spasticity has been an area of considerable growth, attracting wide scientific interest; in contrast, fatigue has received little attention and investment. Yet these symptoms have the potential to impact upon both the efficiency of the rehabilitation programme and its efficacy.

Fatigue

Many people with MS describe the fatigue associated with their condition as an overwhelming sense of tiredness, lack of energy or feeling of exhaustion which is out of all proportion to the level of activity undertaken.

The MS Council for Clinical Practice Guidelines define it as: 'a subjective lack of physical and/or mental energy that is perceived by the individual or care-giver to interfere with usual and desired activities' (Fatigue Guidelines Development Panel Members, 1998). The characteristics of MS fatigue are that:

- It comes on easily
- It prevents physical functioning

- It is worsened by heat
- It interferes with responsibilities and productivity

The advanced practitioner should assess the extent to which fatigue is impacting on the individual's situation and consider:

- If symptoms of depression appear to be coexisting with the fatigue
- If other factors such as disturbed sleep, pain or poor nutrition are contributory factors
- If other medications are exaggerating the fatigue
- How management of the fatigue could be improved

Fatigue is often poorly understood, so education as to the nature of fatigue and its exacerbating factors is an important aspect of the nurse's role.

Assessment should aim to identify any such exacerbating factors – like infection, medication, inappropriate activity patterns and lack of appropriate adaptations/equipment – and attempt to resolve these by appropriate referral for treatment, advice and guidance. As a key worker, the advanced practitioner can support the team to ensure that the planning of any rehabilitation programme takes full account of fatigue management for the individual.

The need to account for the individualised nature of MS is central to successful intervention. Thus for each impairment there is an unwritten first recommendation – 'do not start or modify treatment until all aspects of the individual's clinical situation have been established and understood, and the wishes and expectations of the person with MS have been established' (NICE Guidelines, 2003).

The following case study illustrates just how significant the impact of fatigue was, and how an individualised approach was utilised in the subsequent management.

Case study

Jenny is a young mother of two children. She first met the specialist nurse from the local community rehabilitation team when she was 38 years old and had been diagnosed with MS for 8 years. She had always been a very active mum, and loved to act spontaneously, taking advantage of any nice weather to go out on picnics or to take the dog for a walk. Although she expressed difficulties with mobility, bladder control and pain, her biggest concern was the overwhelming fatigue she experienced on a daily basis. She described being 'wiped out' often for long periods of the day. This prevented her, she felt, from fulfilling her role as wife and mother. As she described the fatigue, she became very tearful and upset. It became clear that much of this distress was due to her perception that people did not either believe or understand how the fatigue could have such a big impact on her life.

Comments made by others led her to believe they considered her to be making too much of it or 'swinging the lead'. She expressed feelings of incredible guilt when her husband, having worked all day, would often have to take over cooking the evening meal and assist in the children's homework and other activities.

Interventions

Assessment: a full assessment of the situation revealed the following exacerbating factors:

- Jenny was struggling up the stairs each time she needed the toilet. The house lacked downstairs facilities and the effort expended in getting up and downstairs left her energy levels depleted.
- Jenny's sleep was often disturbed because of the pain in her left hip.
- She demonstrated high levels of stress due to the time it took undertaking activities for her children and her husband. Making it to school in time to collect her children was a daily worry.
- Jenny's strategy was to get as much as possible done in the morning and then collapse after lunch.

Following long discussions with Jenny and her family, which included information and education on fatigue, a plan was agreed.

Involvement of the occupational therapist within the team to consider appropriate adaptations not only to minimise the need to use the stairs, but to assist with conserving Jenny's energy. This involved both a short- and long-term view to address the immediate problem and to anticipate likely future needs.

The occupational therapist and the team physiotherapist considered Jenny's daily activities and assisted her in identifying a plan that would involve paced activity/exercise and planned rest periods.

The GP was involved with the physiotherapist to assess the pain in her left hip, which was disturbing her sleep. He was also able to rule out any underlying medical condition that may have been contributing to the fatigue and to review her medications in case these were aggravating the situation. The GP together with Jenny and the team also considered the use of amantadine, 200 mg daily, which can offer small clinical benefit in the management of fatigue. This was declined by Jenny.

A referral to the local social services department enabled Jenny to access direct payments to employ her own carer. This gave Jenny the opportunity to receive appropriate care that she could direct according to the priorities that each day brought. By eliminating the pressure to try and keep on top of all the household activities herself, she was able to focus on the most important aspects: being there to collect her children from school, having enough energy to help with homework and other activities, and being awake to spend some time with her husband in the evening.

Jenny and her family initiated a number of other strategies (e.g. internet shopping), which all combined to give a very acceptable outcome to what was initially a major problem.

Spasticity

The term 'spasticity' is often used by health care professionals to collectively describe the unique range of symptoms that can result from a combination of the upper motor neurone syndrome, biochemical changes and/or pain (Jarrett, 2004). It is a common symptom of neurological disease and is frequently experienced by people with MS.

The most common definition used is: 'A motor disorder characterised by a velocity-dependent increase in tonic stretch reflexes (muscle tone) with exaggerated tendon jerks, resulting from hyperexcitability of the stretch reflex, as one component of the upper motor neurone syndrome' (Lance, 1980). In simple terms, if spasticity is present when a limb is passively moved or stretched, the limb will feel stiff. However, this definition, although widely used, does not begin to describe the impact that spasticity can have on the individual. Spasticity can affect physical activities such as walking, transferring, washing, dressing and sexual activity, and can also have an emotional impact on mood, self-image and motivation (Currie, 2001; Porter, 2001). However, spasticity isn't always detrimental and may even have positive consequences for vascular flow, assisting in transfers and even walking (Losseff & Thompson, 1995).

Effective management is often complex and challenging, as spasms can vary from day to day and even hour to hour. Involving members of the rehabilitation team, the individual, their families and any carers, formal or informal, is vital to ensure that appropriate treatment measures are employed. A specialist nurse who may have worked with the individual for long periods, can have detailed knowledge of how spasticity and its management impacts on the client, and is well placed to share this knowledge with other specialists who may become involved in their client's care.

Whilst acknowledging that effective management requires a multidisciplinary approach, this section will focus initially on the role of nurses generally within spasticity management, and then, more specifically, how a nurse consultant led the redesign of a service for patients considering and receiving intrathecal baclofen therapy.

Jarrett (2004) identified eight points on which to base nursing practice and health education:

- Prevention of sensory stimuli
- Postures and positioning
- Moving and handling
- Drug education
- Pain
- Sexual dysfunction

- Emotional issues and depression
- Impact on employment and social activities

The key responsibilities for nurses within these eight points can be summarised under the following headings:

- Prevention
- Education
- Support
- Enablement

Prevention: It is argued that spasticity cannot be prevented. Therefore prevention, in this sense, seeks to encompass a variety of approaches designed to maintain and promote function, minimise pain, maximise comfort and prevent secondary complications. Prevention of sensory stimuli is vital to the effective management of spasticity. Problems can include:

- Red/broken/infected skin
- Pressure ulcers
- Ingrown toe nails
- Tight-fitting orthoses, clothes or Velcro straps from leg bags
- Bladder problems, e.g. infections, incomplete emptying
- Bowel problems, e.g. constipation, impaction, diarrhoea

Nurses have key skills in optimising bladder and bowel function, maintaining skin integrity and maximising hygiene, and are vital to the multidisciplinary team approach.

Postures and positioning: are also key elements to prevent worsening of the condition. Postures in standing, lying and sitting are crucial in managing a person's spasticity and for preventing pain, soft tissue shortening and skin breakdown (Kirkwood & Bardsley, 2001). Within an inpatient or residential setting, nurses often work with individuals throughout a 24-hour period enabling posture and positioning to be assessed at different times. This information can be fed back to members of the multidisciplinary team in order to evaluate the effectiveness of their interventions.

Moving and handling: is linked with posture and positioning. For people with severe spasms this can be complex, and can pose a threat not only to their own safety but to their carers (Jarrett, 2002). A full risk assessment of the situation should be undertaken by appropriate members of the team and recommendations given as to the use of appropriate equipment such as T-rolls, pillows, hoists and sliding boards. Any stretching and standing exercises prescribed by a physiotherapist should be encouraged and facilitated.

Pain: associated with spasticity has been described as a deep, gnawing, constant pain which can be very difficult to treat (Thompson, 1998). Repositioning, physiotherapy and readjustment of seating systems can help to relieve discomfort from malalignment (Jarrett, 2004).

Drugs: antispasticity drugs, such as baclofen, can be helpful. While drugs, like carbamazepine, amitriptyline or gabapentin, can be tried for the relief of symptoms in individuals describing neuropathic pain. Identifying pain, assessing the effectiveness of prescribed treatments and relaying the information back to team members are important aspects of the nurse's role.

Education: The management of spasticity involves an educational component. This is to ensure that the individual understands spasticity as a phenomenon and its potential consequences, thereby optimising compliance with recommendations and engagement in the process. Information regarding treatment options enables the individual to make informed choices in the light of known advantages and disadvantages, effects and side-effects. The education of families, carers and other staff groups provides the opportunity for management to be consistent and ongoing over time and within different settings. Nurses have an important role to play in the education process and have many opportunities for imparting information and sharing knowledge.

Support: The impact of spasticity can be far-reaching, not only on the individual's lifestyle but also that of their families and carers (Porter, 2001). It can also affect how an individual perceives him/herself and how others perceive them, which can, in turn, lead to low mood, low self-esteem, frustration and poor self-image Spasms can also make normal sexual behaviour difficult, and this may impair the individual's ability to establish or maintain partnership relations. Nurses can provide much needed support to individuals and their families to cope with the emotional and psychological impact of spasticity. They are well placed to signpost them to other professionals and organisations for information, support and interventions, including: counsellors, psychologists and specialists with particular expertise in sexual problems associated with neurological disease.

Enablement: The extent of an individual's spasticity and spasms may mean the person requires assistance with some or all of the activities of daily living. Nurses should enable individuals to develop appropriate coping strategies, and to manage their own abilities/limitations so that input from professionals is kept to a minimum, allowing them to get on with their lives as much as possible. Although the locus of control should be with the individual, the team should be there to support choice whenever possible and appropriate.

The management of spasticity can be a rewarding challenge for health care professionals in any health or social setting. Interventions can range from exercise and stretches through to more invasive procedures, like the use of botulinum toxin and intrathecal baclofen therapy.

Continuous intrathecal baclofen

Continuous intrathecal baclofen infusion is an effective treatment option in the management of severe spasticity of either cerebral or spinal origin (Trent Institute for Health Services Research, 2000).

Severe spasticity is a significant problem for many patients with spinal cord injury, multiple sclerosis and acquired brain injury, causing a loss of independence and mobility, pain, sleep problems, difficulties in nursing care and aggravation of other problems such as skin breakdown and urinary incontinence.

Intrathecal baclofen (ITB) therapy is used in the treatment of patients whose spasticity is refractory to other treatments (including physical therapies and oral treatments) or who experience unacceptable side-effects with oral drug therapy. As the dosage of baclofen administered in this way is so low (micrograms), side-effects associated with taking it orally are minimised.

Baclofen is administered intrathecally via a subcutaneously implanted electronic pump with a reservoir and catheter. The pump is usually placed in an abdominal pocket fashioned in either the left or right abdominal quadrant. The tip of the catheter is placed at the level of the second or third lumbar vertebrae, or higher. This system is then electronically programmed using a computer and telemetry, allowing different dose regimes to be delivered.

The use of ITB is not without risk. Minimising complications and maximising therapeutic benefit requires a coordinated approach from an experienced team including:

- Neurologist
- Consultant in rehabilitation medicine
- Neurosurgeon
- Nurse
- Physiotherapist
- Occupational therapist

Development and redesign of ITB therapy

A literature review undertaken to support the service redesign, resulted in the following key findings:

- ITB therapy: requires a coordinated approach by an experienced team. A comprehensive multidisciplinary strategy is required that minimises risks whilst maximising therapeutic benefit and which incorporates clearly defined goals.
- Patient selection: ITB therapy is effective in carefully selected patients.
- Outcome measures:
    — Ashworth score was by far the most consistent measure employed for recording spasticity, particularly pre- and post-test dose.
    — the Function Independence Measure (FIM) score is highly significant in measuring functional change in patients with spasticity of spinal origin.
    — qualitative measures are needed to relate patient goals to treatment.

- Research: a need for more qualitative research was identified, with respect to body image, impact on lifestyle and function and quality of life for patients and carers.
- Risks: adverse effects:
  — overdose of ITB was widely reported, with resulting respiratory depression requiring ventilatory support.
  — tolerance and dose increases occur with prolonged use.
- Patient stories: analysis of patient stories identified the need for:
  — a flexible and responsive service
  — rapid access for problem-solving
  — readily available expertise
  — a support group
  — comprehensive information and education

Patients and carers were invited to join the Service Redesign Project Group by personal letter and by a follow-up telephone call. Some expressed reservations due to the large contingency of medical personnel in the project group, which was slightly intimidating for them. At their suggestion, an informal gathering was held for two hours when the participants were informed of progress to date and were asked to contribute their ideas, comments and opinions on any aspect of the service. Notes were taken of this meeting, with their permission, and the key suggestions were as follows:

- To provide patients with the opportunity to meet with someone who already has an ITB pump fitted, prior to their own implantation.
- To set up a register of patients with ITB pumps who would be willing to meet prospective patients.
- To set up a support group that would meet every six months for informal support, discussions, education and exchange of news.
- Patient information leaflets to include a list of minor problems that could occur after surgery.
- To exchange details, re: websites of interest.

In summary, they were overwhelmingly in support of a dedicated specialist clinic. However, they wished the service provider to consider ease of access and flexibility. For example, if alterations were made to the drug dosage and it proved to be unsuitable, patients would not wish to wait a month until the next clinic but would wish to be offered an interim appointment. This would need to be accommodated within a general rehabilitation clinic or by individual appointments with the nurse consultant or clinical nurse specialist. Domiciliary visits would need to be retained for those unable to travel.

Future involvement of patients and carers: The following suggestions were made to ensure the continued involvement of patients and carers:

- Information from the six-monthly support group to be fed back to the Baclofen Services Forum. This was a forum where health care professionals involved in the management of ITB met to network, discuss clinical practices/case studies and suggest areas for research and service improvement.
- Patients and carers were to be invited to the Baclofen Services Forum.
- One-to-one interviews to be undertaken to address gaps in the evidence base, e.g. body image, impact on lifestyle and psychological impact.
- Patients and carers to be involved in the audit of the service.
- All comments/complaints to be analysed, with feedback to the service via the Baclofen Services Forum.

Outcome measures: The Project Group discussed this in detail. It was agreed that specific outcome measures would be adopted for all patients, in line with the evidence base for specific aspects of the care pathway:

- Modified Ashworth Scale for recording severity of spasticity.
- Visual analogue for scoring pain associated with spasticity.
- Spasm Frequency Scale for determining frequency of spasms per day.
- Use of video recording pre- and post-implantation, with patient consent to visually demonstrate the effects of treatment.
- Achievement of client goals to be documented and audited to establish if expectations of treatment were met, plus satisfaction with treatment outcomes.
- Comments/complaints related to the service to be discussed at the Baclofen Services Forum to influence service development and delivery.
- Problems experienced with individual patients to be discussed and used for training and education purposes via the Baclofen Services Forum/ training days. Patient confidentiality to be maintained at all times.
- Monitoring of waiting lists, referrals, transitional arrangements and patient satisfaction surveys to also provide information in order to demonstrate effectiveness of the service from both the patient and the service provider's perspective.

Risks and risk management: Table 9.5 demonstrates the potential risks associated with ITB therapy and how the process of service redesign attempted to address these risks.

Any incidents/near misses would be reported in accordance with policies and procedures. A database would include a record of incidents to enable monitoring and appropriate action. Quarterly training sessions would be arranged to which all staff involved in ITB therapy would be invited. A record of attendance and evaluation forms would be completed.

Conclusions

This chapter has attempted to capture the very essence of nursing in neuro-rehabilitation. The spectrum of possibilities for advanced nursing roles, from the post-acute management of traumatic injury through to the long-term management of progressive disease, have been identified and described.

As a specialty, neurorehabilitation has been considered in terms of both the challenges and opportunities that it provides to practitioners working within the field. Both authors have worked as nurse consultants in this area and hope to have weaved their enthusiasm for the subject area into the chapter, as well as those values and beliefs fundamental to the delivery of rehabilitation practice that is attuned to the individual's needs.

The future for neurorehabilitation will no doubt bring many more challenges and opportunities as people live longer, technology advances and individuals with severe injuries and disabilities experience increased chances of survival. The agendas around public health, chronic disease management and choice also need to be incorporated into practice as the emphasis moves from illness to health, and the power and control shifts from the practitioner to the patient. The opportunity to advance nursing roles has never been greater, and neurorehabilitation offers immense potential for those advanced roles. It is a specialised field of practice that: utilises many skills; fine tunes problem-solving techniques; embraces all age groups; allows for the transfer of previous experience and knowledge; incorporates interdisciplinary team working; stimulates learning; and offers many, many more opportunities and experiences.

References

Barnes N. and Radermacher H. (2003) *Community Rehabilitation in Neurology.* Cambridge, Cambridge University Press, p. 25.

British Society of Rehabilitation Medicine (1998) *Rehabilitation after Traumatic Brain Injury.* London, BSRM Publications.

British Society of Rehabilitation Medicine and Royal College of Physicians (2003) *Rehabilitation Following Acquired Brain Injury: National Clinical Guidelines.* London, RCP & BSRM Publications.

Burgess M. (2002) *Multiple Sclerosis Theory and Practice for Nurses.* London, Whurr Publishers.

UK Multiple Sclerosis Specialist Nurse Association, Multiple Sclerosis Trust (2003) *Competencies for MS Specialist Nurses.* London, Royal College of Nursing.

Currie R. (2001) Spasticity: a common symptom of multiple sclerosis. *Nursing Standard,* **15** (33), 47–52.

Department of Health (1993) *A Vision for the Future: The Nursing, Midwifery and Health Visiting Contribution to Health and Health Care.* London, HMSO.

Department of Health (1999) *Making a Difference: Strengthening the Nursing, Midwifery and Health Visiting Contribution to Health and Health Care.* London, HMSO.

Department of Health (2001) *Government Response to the Health Select Committee: Third Report. Head Injury Rehabilitation.* London, HMSO.

Department of Health (2002) *Liberating the Talents: Helping Primary Care Trusts and Nurses to Deliver the NHS Plan.* London, HMSO.

Department of Health (2004) *Chronic Disease Management.* London, DH.

Fatigue Guidelines Development Panel Members (1998) *Fatigue and Multiple Sclerosis Evidence Based Management Strategies for Fatigue in Multiple Sclerosis. Multiple Sclerosis Council for Clinical Practice Guidelines.* Washington D.C., Paralysed Veterans of America.

Fleminger S. (2003) Managing agitation and aggression after head injury. *British Medical Journal*, **327**, 4–5.

Hardy K. (2002) Shaping the NSF for Long Term Conditions: The Views of Service Users, Carers and Voluntary Organisations. Long-Term Medical Conditions Alliance and the Neurological Alliance.

Holland N. and Halper J. (1999) Primary care management of MS. *Advance for Nurse Practitioners*, March, 1–8.

Jarrett L. (2002) *Care Pathway: The Role of the Nurse in the Management of Spasticity.* Letchworth, MS Trust.

Jarrett L. (2004) The role of the nurse in the management of spasticity. *Nursing and Residential Care*, **6** (3), 116–119.

Kay A.D. and Teasdale G.M. (2001) Head injury in the UK. *World Journal of Surgery*, **25**, Part 9, 1210–1220.

Kirkwood C. and Bardsley G.I. (2001) Seating and positioning in spasticity. In: *Upper Motor Neurone Syndrome and Spasticity. Clinical Management and Neurophysiology* (M. Barnes and G. Johnson, eds). Cambridge, Cambridge University Press.

Kraft G.H., Freal J.E. and Coryell J.K. (1986) Disability, disease duration, and rehabilitation service needs in multiple sclerosis: patient perspectives. *Archives of Physical Medicine and Rehabilitation*, **67** (3), 164–168. [Cited in: Burgess, M. (2002) *Multiple Sclerosis Theory and Practice for Nurses.* London, Whurr Publishers, p. 75.]

Lance J.W. (1980) Symposium synopsis. In: *Spasticity: Disordered Motor Control* (R.G. Fieldman, R.R. Young and W.P. Koella, eds). Chicago, Year Book Medical Publishers, pp. 485–494.

Losseff N. and Thompson A.J. (1995) The medical management of increased tone. *Physiotherapy*, **81** (8), 480–484.

McMillan T. and Ledder H. (2001) A survey of services provided by community neuro rehabilitations teams in South East England. *Clinical Rehabilitation*, **15**, 582–588.

Miller J., Pentland B. and Berrol A. (1990) Early evaluation and management. In: *Rehabilitation of the Adult and Child with Traumatic Brain Injury*, 2nd edn (Rosenthan M., Griffith E., Bond M. and Miller J., eds). Philadelphia, F.A. Davis Co.

Murray C.J. and Lopez A.D. (1997) Alternative projections of mortality and disability by cause 1990–2020: Global Burden of Disease Study. *Lancet*, **349** (9064), 1498–1504.

National Institute for Clinical Excellence (2003) *Clinical Guideline 8. Multiple Sclerosis. Management of Multiple Sclerosis in Primary and Secondary Care.* London, NICE, p. 26.

Neurological Alliance (2003) *Neuro Numbers.* Review published in London by the Neuro Alliance in conjunction with the British Association of Neurological Surgeons and Royal College of Nursing.

Oxtoby M. (1999) A team approach to neurological disease. In: *Patient Care in Neurology* (A.C. Williams, ed.). Oxford, Oxford University Press, pp. 433–441.

Pickard J., Seeley H., Kirker S., Maimaris C., McGlashan K., Roeis E. and Greenwood R. (2004) Mapping rehabilitation resources for head injury. *Journal of the Royal Society of Medicine*, **97**, 384–389.

Porter B. (2001) Nursing management of spasticity. *Primary Health Care*, **11** (1), 25–29.

Powell T. (1994) Head Injury – A Practical Guide. Bicester, Oxfordshire, Speechmark Publications Ltd for Headway.

RCS (1999) RCS Guidelines: Report of The Working Party on the Management of Patients with Head Injuries. London, RCSENG Communications, p. 33.

Rosenthal M., Griffith E., Bond M. and Miller J. (eds) (1990) *Rehabilitation of the Adult and Child with Traumatic Brain Injury*, 2nd edn. Philadelphia, F.A. Davis Co.

Russell R. (1932) Cerebral involvement in head injury. *Brain*, **55**, 549.

Sirois M.J., Lavoie A. and Dionne C. (2004) Impact of transfer delays to rehabilitation in patients with severe trauma. *Archives of Physical Medicine and Rehabilitation*, **85** (2), 184–191.

Smith P. (1992) *The Emotional Labour of Nursing*. London, Macmillan.

Thompson, A.J. (1998) Spasticity rehabilitation: a rational approach to clinical management. In: *Spasticity Rehabilitation* (G. Sheean, ed.). London, Churchill Communications.

Thornhill S., Teasdale M., Murray G., McEwen J., Roy C. and Penny K. (2000) Disability in young people and adults one year after head injury: prospective cohort study. *British Medical Journal*, **320**, 1631–1635.

Trent Institute for Health Services Research (2000) *The Effectiveness of Intrathecal Baclofen in the Management of Patients with Severe Spasticity*. Nottingham, TIHSR.

Turner-Stokes L., Williams A. and Abraham R. (2001) Clinical standards for specialist community rehabilitation services in the UK. *Clinical Rehabilitation*, **15**, 611–623.

World Health Organization (2002) *Innovative Care for Chronic Conditions; Building Blocks for Action*. Geneva, WHO, WHO/MNC/CCH/02.01, www.who.int/ncd/chronic-care/index.htm

Chapter 10
Supporting People with Long-term Conditions

Rebecca Jester

Introduction

The aim of this chapter is to critically discuss new ways of working to support patients with chronic long-term conditions and, specifically, the implementation of case management in the UK. The chapter also presents an overview of self-management, which is crucial to the success of providing coordinated and integrated care. There is discussion on the importance of how specialist nurses in rehabilitation and case managers will need to liaise closely to fully exploit their collective expertise in the care and management of patients with long-term conditions, and to avoid fragmented care and duplication of effort. Indicative content within this chapter includes:

- Background to new ways of working with people with chronic long-term conditions
- Implementation of case management
- Models of assessment for clients with long-term conditions
- Single assessment process
- Preparation for self-management
- Medicines' management
- The interplay of specialist/advanced nurses and case managers
- The role of the expert patient
- Case study to exemplify new ways of working

Background

Some 17.5 million people in the UK report living with a long-term condition (LTC) (DH, 2005), while chronic disease affects more than 100 million Americans, accounting for half of total health care costs (Redman, 2004). Many of these people suffer with more than one long-term condition and experience significant pain, disability and distress on a daily basis. The magnitude of the

Table 10.1 Key factors underpinning new ways of working.

• Empowerment of patients toward self-management and self-efficacy
• Integrated working between health, social and voluntary services to provide seamless care and minimise duplication of effort
• Proactive approaches to chronic disease management; greater emphasis on early detection and minimisation of related complications
• Improved communication and informatics between service providers: integrated care pathways, patient-held records, compatible IT systems
• Dramatic improvement in medicines' management
• Service provision built upon mutual trust and respect of one another's contribution to the management of patients with long-term conditions.

problem is exemplified by the fact that people aged 60 and over have an average of 2.2 chronic conditions. Unfortunately, a predominantly biomedical approach to the management of people with LTCs has led to a fragmented service provision that is reactive, unplanned and episodic. This model of service provision has resulted in frequent unplanned admissions to secondary care, with 5% of inpatients, many with an LTC, accounting for 42% of all acute hospital bed days (DH, 2005). It has been predicted that, to sustain the current level and model of service provision for people with an LTC, every school leaver in 2015 would need to be recruited into the health care professions. Clearly, this is not feasible and in the context of an increasingly aged and sick society new ways of working need to be developed.

The Public Health White Paper *Choosing Health* sets out the Government's strategy for supporting people with LTCs in the UK. Furthermore, the Government has set specific targets to improve outcomes for people with long-term conditions through the public service agreement (PSA). The specific targets of the PSA are to:

- Reduce inpatient emergency bed days by 5% by March 2008 (compared to 2003/2004 figures).
- Offer a personalised care plan for vulnerable people most at risk.

A significant change in the model of service provision for people with long-term conditions is needed to achieve these targets. New ways of working must be underpinned by a number of key factors, which are outlined in Table 10.1.

The NHS and Social Care Long Term Conditions Model aims to embrace all the factors detailed in Table 10.1 and lead to an improved quality of life for LTC patients and a more effective use of resources. The NHS model builds upon the Kaiser Permanente triangle of classification of management of LTCs, which has been widely implemented across the USA. The Kaiser Permanente triangle classifies the management of LTCs into three levels as follows:

- Level 1: 70–80% of the target population require self-care support/ management

- Level 2: high risk – requires disease/care management
- Level 3: high complexity – requires case management

A key element to this model is the role of the case manager, which is discussed below.

Case management

Case management encompasses not only the evidence-based management of specific diseases, but also the holistic care needs of the individual. The Department of Health has outlined a number of key steps in implementing case management:

Step 1 – Identifying the most vulnerable patients
Step 2 – Developing the community matron role
Step 3 – Carrying out thorough assessment and care planning
Step 4 – Coordinating care and services

Step 1 – Identifying the most vulnerable patients

This requires high levels of collaborative working between health and social care services in both primary and secondary care to accurately identify those patients most at risk. Several approaches should be adopted, including: analysis of patients' health records; and discussion with key professionals currently involved with the client, e.g. GPs, specialists in secondary care. This requires robust informatics systems, which are compatible across the primary and secondary health care sectors. Unfortunately, at the time of writing this is not the case, which has therefore necessitated most of the information being gleaned from individual health care professionals. As specialist nurses within rehabilitation we have a key role in supporting the accurate identification of the most vulnerable patients. To do this we must have an understanding of the criteria for case management. Although there is some degree of variation in the criteria between strategic health authorities, most agree that patients with three or more chronic long-term conditions who have had two or more unplanned hospital admissions within a 12-month period meet the criteria.

Take time now to reflect on how many of your patients meet these criteria and if they are currently being case-managed. It is likely that in the early phases of implementation some of your patients will not have been included and you will need to bring them to the attention of the primary care trust responsible for organising case management.

Step 2 – Developing the community matron role

There has been a lack of consistency surrounding the titles and roles associated with case management in the UK. Many areas have appointed community matrons to take on the role; most of these posts require a community nursing background. However, some SHAs have adopted a more flexible approach to the role and have encouraged individuals from different health professional backgrounds, such as occupational therapists, community pharmacists, etc., to take up posts as case managers. As specialist nurses working with rehabilitation patients we have a duty to develop an in-depth understanding of the case manager role, and to develop strong relationships and clear channels of communication with them to promote seamless care delivery to patients and avoid duplication of effort and waste of resources.

Take some time now to identify case managers in your local area and discuss strategies to maximise collaborative working with your colleagues.

Step 3 – Carrying out thorough assessment and care planning

The case manager is responsible for conducting a thorough holistic needs-based assessment of the client. This should be done in partnership with the client and informal carers, as appropriate. The holistic assessment of clients requiring case management is complex, and therefore requires the application of an appropriate framework to provide structure, logical sequencing, a reduced risk of missing valuable information and the avoidance of repetition. Depending on the level of support required, i.e. level 1–3, the framework will need to be responsive to a continuum of support, ranging from a framework based on self-management, health beliefs, health behaviours and strong educational component to a framework with a stronger biomedical focus and based on national service and quality and outcomes frameworks. However, for all levels the framework must be multidisciplinary and multiagency and avoid repetition of assessment.

Appropriate theoretical frameworks that engender the key aims of self-management and empowerment of the client should underpin the assessment. The traditional biomedical model of patient assessment (based upon a review of body systems) will be insufficient to capture all the data needed to develop a holistic plan of managed care. Table 10.2 provides a summary of a number of assessment frameworks that lend themselves to chronic disease management, because they focus on the client's ability to cope and adapt with changes in their lives due to chronic disease/s and are based upon concepts of health, well being and independence. It is not possible within this chapter to critically review each of these models, but further recommended reading is provided at the end of this chapter.

Below, an overview of the single assessment process (SAP) is provided as a multiagency model, which minimises repetition of assessment.

The single assessment process

The single assessment process (SAP) was developed as a practical lever toward a model of integrated health and social care and achieving the genuinely

Table 10. 2 Summary of frameworks of assessment suitable for patients with long-term conditions.

Model of assessment	Author	Summary of key points
Typology of 11 functional health patterns	Gordon (1987)	Based upon 11 health patterns: health perception/health management; nutritional–metabolic; elimination; activity–exercise; cognitive–perceptual; sleep–rest; self-perception/self-concept; role-relationship; sexuality–reproductive; coping/stress-tolerance; and value-belief.
Maslow's 'Hierarchy of Needs'	Maslow (1987)	Based upon a hierarchy of an individual's needs beginning with physiological, then safety and security followed by love and belonging, then esteem and self-esteem and, finally, self-actualisation.
Wellness framework	Pinnell & de Meneses (1986)	Based upon five aspects of well being: degree of fitness; level of nutrition; sensitivity to the environment; risk appraisal and level of life stress; and lifestyle and personal health habits.
Orem's Self-Care Model	Orem (1984)	Based upon three domains of self-care requisites: universal aspects, including physiological and normalcy; developmental stages of human development and factors that impinge upon; and health deviation, concordance to treatment/advice and lifestyle modification to improve health.
Neuman's Systems Model of Assessment	Neuman (1982)	Focuses on the impact on both the patient and the caregiver and is based upon stressors and strengths perceived by both parties. Identifies a number of factors to be considered, which include intrapersonal, interpersonal and extrapersonal.
Roy's Adaptation Model	Roy (1984)	Based upon modes of adaptation, which include: physiological, role function, self-concept and interdependence modes.

person-centred care and integrated services envisaged in the *National Service Framework for Older People* (DH, 2001a). The aim of the Single Assessment Process, delivering person-centred care, is:

'to ensure that older people's needs are assessed and evaluated fully, with professionals sharing information appropriately and not repeating assessments already carried out by others. This requires a high degree of mutual trust, robust systems for information-sharing, and a clear understanding of respective roles and responsibilities.' (DH, 2004a)

The purpose of SAP is to ensure that older people receive appropriate, effective and timely responses to their health and social care needs, and that professional resources are used effectively. In pursuit of these aims, SAP should ensure that:

- Individuals are placed at the heart of assessment and care planning, and these processes are timely and in proportion to an individual's needs.
- Professionals are willing, able and confident to use their judgement.
- Care plans or statements of service delivery are routinely produced and service users receive a copy.
- Professionals contribute to assessments in the most effective way, and care coordinators are agreed in individual cases when necessary.
- Information is collected, stored and shared as effectively as possible and subject to consent.
- Professionals and agencies do not duplicate each other's assessments.

The Department of Health set an implementation milestone for the SAP of 1st April 2005. However, many organisations have struggled to meet this target. This is exemplified by the West Midlands SAP Cross Boundary Project (2004), which evaluated progress on the implementation of SAP across the West Midlands region. Findings illustrated a wide discrepancy between trusts in the following areas:

- Format and type of assessment documentation (mostly still paper-based)
- Person-held records – where available had differing content and format
- Contact assessment – differing demographic data collected

As specialist nurses in rehabilitation it is important to develop a good understanding of the SAP and to ensure that we encourage patients to bring their person-held record to any appointment or visit related to their rehabilitation. We also need to ensure that other members of the rehabilitation multidisciplinary team familiarise themselves with the document and record their assessment findings, interventions and evaluations in the patient's person-held document. This will assist case managers and other community colleagues to be up-to-date with the rehabilitation goals of the client and be able to contribute effectively toward attainment of these goals.

Step 3 of case management not only involves assessment, but also the development of care plans. An integrated care pathway (ICP) should be developed to promote interdisciplinary and multiagency working and a client-centred approach. Many professionals working in rehabilitation will be well versed in the development, implementation and evaluation of various ICPs. They provide a medium for interdisciplinary working and should encompass the patient journey from primary to secondary care and back again (please see Chapter 1 for discussion on ICPs). Care planning for patients with long-term conditions needs to address the transition from active treatment to palliative care. There has been significant development in end-of-life pathways in the UK in recent years, aiming to provide consistent high-quality approaches to end-of-life care, including timely recognition by health care professionals when the emphasis of care needs to be changed. For this to be implemented fully there must be strong working relationships and clearly identified channels of communication and referral between case managers, specialist nurses in rehabilitation and palliative care teams.

Step 4 – Coordinating care and services

The community matron/case manager has a pivotal role in coordinating care and services. They must ensure that the client and their informal carer/s are actively involved in all areas of decision-making relating to their care. Rapid and easy access to clinical investigations and their results is essential if case management is to work effectively. There will need to be effective liaison between the case manager role and the specialist nurse in rehabilitation to ensure the client goes to the right setting for their continued recuperation and rehabilitation.

Now take the opportunity to review the current systems of liaison and collaborative working between the rehabilitation team and local case managers within your organisation to ensure that patients' care is coordinated and seamless.

Preparation for self-management

Self-management of chronic disease is engendered both within the public service agreement targets and case management. However, the transition to a model of self-management for patients with LTCs, their families and health care professionals will take time and careful preparation. Over time, many people with long-term conditions have developed learned helpless (Seligman, 1975) and an external locus of control about their health (Rotter, 1966). This has been perpetuated by a paternalistic model of health care delivery, despite the importance of patient participation and control over their care and treatment at an individual and societal level being highlighted in recent years (Aronson, 1999; Mullen & Spurgeon, 2000). Redman (2004) suggests that living with a chronic disease/s creates three types of work for patients:

- Work necessitated by the disease, such as taking medicine and maintaining therapeutic exercise regimens.
- Work of maintaining everyday life, such as employment and family.
- Work of dealing with an altered view of the future, including changing life plans (grief process).

Preparation of clients for self-management (SM) requires a considerable investment of both time and resources if they are to gain the skills and develop the confidence to use both diagnostic and therapeutic techniques to manage their health effectively (Partridge & Hill, 2002). Formalised SM preparation programmes are required, which may be disease-specific, but typically can include several types of disease as many of the skills required are generic. Redman (2004) suggests that SM programmes must use problem-based learning approaches and include the following key elements:

- Skill development in problem-solving
- Development of clinical judgement
- Self-efficacy building
- Belief modification and symptom reinterpretation

   The last point emphasises the importance of clients learning to accept that their condition is not curable, is not due to something they have done wrong and is controllable by them in partnership with health care professionals, as then they are much more likely to be successful in self-management. Didactic methods of information delivery are unlikely to achieve SM. Rather, psychoeducational techniques that help to foster problem analysis and option appraisal are needed, such as problem-based learning using relevant worked examples and scenarios. There is a need to adopt blended approaches to SM preparation, including group sessions, individual learning plans and the use of web-based material, as appropriate. Clearly, individual entry knowledge and experience, social and cultural background, levels of formal education and psychological status need to be taken into consideration. All of this preparation must be spread over a prolonged period and be regularly updated and monitored to facilitate mastery by the client in the skills of SM, so they can be recalled readily when the client is experiencing stress and/or exacerbation of symptoms. Preparation for SM programmes is also highly relevant to informal carers of clients in rehabilitation or to those being case managed.

Medicines' management

For a number of years it has been identified that patients with chronic long-term conditions are often poorly managed in terms of their medicines. Frequently, patients are unsure of what they are supposed to take, when and why, which often results in poor compliance with prescription medicines. To date, there has been no systematic approach to reviewing patients' medication. This, combined with burgeoning pharmaceutical costs, has necessitated the Department of Health to drive forward a systematic approach to medicines' management both within primary and secondary care (DH, 2004b). The principles of medicines' management have been summarised as follows (DH, 2004b):

- Involving patients in the choice of treatment
- Monitoring for benefits and safety
- Deciding whether a medicine is needed
- Reviewing effectiveness of treatment
- Deciding when to stop treatment

- Reducing medicines' wastage
- Identifying over- and undertreatment
- Making best use of resources: evidence-based formularies and guidelines
- Better communications between prescribers, patients and carers
- Providing patient-centred information
- Consideration of non-pharmacological options, such as advice, health promotion, etc.

It is imperative that it is clear who will undertake a patient's medicines' review and how often this is carried out. Also, that changes made to medications are clearly communicated between primary and secondary health care professionals. Polypharmacy has been identified as a significant risk factor in precipitating falls and that it can have other severe deleterious effects on patients' health. Specialist nurses in rehabilitation and nurses involved in supporting patients with chronic diseases in the community must work collaboratively to implement and effectively evaluate medicines' management in this vulnerable client group.

The interplay of specialist/advanced nurses and case managers

Many of us working in specialist/advanced roles within rehabilitation will be concerned about how our expertise and knowledge of the client will be used in the context of case management. The very nature of specialisation can lead to a reductionist approach to viewing the management of the client. However, since many of our patients have comorbid conditions to contend with, the need to view them holistically is the reason many of us developed our roles to fill a gap created by specialisation of medicine. For example, many patients with severe osteoarthritis or a hip fracture have congestive heart failure and diabetes. It is important that, as specialist nurses, we take the lead in establishing firm partnerships and clear channels of communication with case managers in our area. It will require tremendous collaborative effort to move toward the target of seamless, coordinated and integrated care. Relatively simple steps, such as encouraging clients to bring their person-held documents to consultations and writing up the summary for their case managers to refer to, will all help toward this goal. Strong collaborative effort between specialist nurses and case managers is essential to minimise unnecessary unplanned hospital admissions and to facilitate efficient and safe discharge from hospital.

The role of the expert patient

The move toward new ways of working in chronic disease management requires a major shift in how services are organised and a significant change in emphasis from the patient merely being a recipient of health and social care to being a valuable resource in their own management. The Department of Health proposed a number of initiatives aimed at maximising the resource of the expert patient, based on the premise that those living with long-term conditions have a wealth of knowledge and experience about coping with their condition/s and that this should be tapped to maximise their own self-management and to support others with similar conditions (DH, 2001b). The model is based on the work of Professor Loring of Stanford University, California, and the success of the Chronic Disease Self-management Program (CDSMP) in the USA. The CDSMP is a highly structured programme led by trained volunteers who are themselves living with a long-term condition. Although, some of the programmes are condition-specific, such as 'Challenge arthritis', a self-management programme for manic depression and self-management in multiple sclerosis, there are a number of generic core topics, including:

- Pain management
- Stress and coping
- Symptom recognition and management
- Problem-solving
- Communicating with professionals

The Department of Health's vision for Expert Patient Programme is to: increase the number of people with chronic disease improving, remaining stable or deteriorating more slowly; promote greater self-management of symptoms by patients; reduce incapacity, specifically in relation to fatigue and sleep deprivation; increase the number of patients retaining or gaining employment; and foster greater empowerment and self-esteem for patients with LTCs. The success of the expert patient initiative will depend on effective collaboration between health care professionals and leading patient representative bodies, and that the approach is consistent with the principles of the NSF for long-term health conditions. Also, there will need to be adequate resources and support available to prepare expert patients and the role of the programme leaders. Many of us working within rehabilitation will already have strong relationships with voluntary organisations and patient groups that can be built upon to develop the role of the expert patient and to set up self-management programmes.

Case study to exemplify new ways of working

Ken, aged 78, with severe osteoarthritis of his hip, that was severely impacting on his quality of life, had been listed for a right total hip replacement by the orthopaedic consultant surgeon. Several weeks later he was asked to attend the specialist nurse-led health maintenance clinic within the acute trust for an assessment of his medical status. This was to ensure he was fit for surgery/ anaesthesia and to provide him with information about his forthcoming procedure, care and rehabilitation. During this consultation it became apparent that Ken was suffering with several comorbid conditions, besides his osteoarthritis, including hypertension and heart failure. He was obese with a body mass index of 35, BP of 160/100 mm/Hg, was short of breath even on mild exertion and had very swollen feet and ankles. A full assessment of the situation revealed the following main exacerbating factors:

- Ken was being prescribed over eight different types of medicines; he was not concordant with taking them because he was unsure what they were for. Their side-effects included severe constipation and frequency and urgency of micturition.
- Ken didn't know that he should be having his blood pressure checked regularly and found getting to the GP surgery very difficult.
- Ken realised he was becoming more obese, but felt that it was impossible to lose weight because of his very limited mobility.
- He was very anxious that he might not be able to have his hip replacement because of his other medical problems, and so hadn't discussed them with the surgeon.

After discussion with Ken and his wife, the orthopaedic ANP contacted Ken's GP and it was decided that Ken would benefit from assessment by one of the local community matrons. Following comprehensive assessment at home by the community matron, Ken was classified as Level 2 within the Kaiser Permanente model and needed disease/care management. The following actions were agreed in partnership with Ken and his wife:

- A full review of his medications to be undertaken. This resulted in fewer medications and improved concordance as Ken was informed fully about what he was taking and why, their potential side-effects and how they could be managed.
- Ken's BP to be regularly monitored by the community nursing team and to be informed about lifestyle modification by the community matron.
- One of the local expert patient programmes to be introduced, specifically for arthritis.
- Ken to be given patient-held records, which he was to bring along to all hospital visits.

As a result of the partnership between primary and secondary care and the intervention of the community matron, Ken became more empowered and in control of his situation. He felt part of the team working toward optimising his general health in preparation for his forthcoming hip replacement and improving his quality of life in the medium and long term. Ken experienced more effective pain relief and a reduction in his breathlessness. Subsequently, he was able to be more active, which contributed to his steady weight loss, and his BP was reduced to within a safe level for surgery/anaesthesia.

Conclusions

This chapter has attempted to discuss some of the key issues related to new ways of working with clients who have long-term chronic disease. The necessity of the successful implementation of case management is reinforced by both the magnitude of the prevalence of chronic disease in contemporary society and the need to support and prepare clients and their families to self-manage their health. However, the importance of adequate SM preparation has to be emphasised if we are to see significant changes in patient empowerment and self-efficacy. Throughout the chapter, the need for close liaison and clear communication channels between specialist nurses and case managers has been affirmed to ensure that our collective expertise is used to its maximum effect.

References

Aronson E. (1999) *The Social Animal*, 8th edn. California, Worth Publishers.

Department of Health (2001a) *National Service Framework for Older People*. London, DH.

Department of Health (2001b) T*he Expert Patient: A New Approach to Chronic Disease Management for the 21st Century*. London, DH.

Department of Health (2004a) *Chronic Disease Management: A Compendium of Information*. London, DH.

Department of Health (2004b) *Management of Medicines – a Resource to Support Implementation of the Wider Aspects of Medicines Management for the National Service Frameworks for Diabetes, Renal Services and Long-Term Conditions*. London, DH.

Department of Health (2005) *Supporting People with Long Term Conditions: An NHS and Social Care Model to Support Local Innovation and Integration*. Leeds, DH.

Gordon M. (1987) *Nursing Diagnosis: Process and Application*, 2nd edn. St Louis, Mosby.

Maslow A. (1987) *Motivation and Personality*, 3rd edn. London, Harper & Row.

Mullen P. and Spurgeon P. (2000) *Priority Setting and the Public*. Abingdon, Radcliffe Medical Press.

Neuman B. (1982) *The Neuman Systems Model*. Norwalk, N.J., Appleton-Century Crofts.

Orem D. (1984) *Nursing: Concepts of Practice*. 2nd edn. New York, McGraw-Hill.

Partridge M. and Hill S. (2002) Enhancing care for people with asthma: the role of communication, education, training and self-management. *European Respiratory Journal*, **16**, 333–348.

Pinnell N. and De Meneses M. (1986) *The Nursing Process: Theory, Application and Related Processes*. Norwalk, N.J., Appleton-Lange.

Redman B. (2004) *Patient Self-Management of Chronic Disease: The Health Care Provider's Challenge*. London, Jones and Bartlett.

Rotter J. (1966) Generalised expectancies for internal versus external control of reinforcement. *Psychological Monographs*, **80**, 1–28.

Roy C. (1984) *Introduction to Nursing: An Adaptation Model*, 2nd edn. Englewood Cliffs, N.J., Prentice Hall.

Seligman M. (1975) *Helplessness: On Depression, Development and Death*. San Francisco, W.H. Freeman.

West Midlands Regional Single Assessment Process Group (2004) *The Single Assessment Process and Cross Boundary Working. A Report Sponsored by the DH – Health & Social Care Change Agent Team.*

Further reading

Pitts M. and Phillips K. (1998) *The Psychology of Health: An Introduction*, 2nd edn. London, Routledge.

Redman B. (2004) *Patient Self-Management of Chronic Disease: The Health Care Provider's Challenge*. London, Jones and Bartlett.

Wakley G. and Chambers R. (2005) *Chronic Disease Management in Primary Care*. Abingdon, Radcliffe Publishing.

Chapter 11
Rehabilitation of Patients with Spinal Cord Injury

Nicki Bellinger

Introduction

Patients with a spinal cord injury (SCI) require rehabilitation of the highest standard to enable them to recover from this life-threatening injury, which presents a major life-changing event for the patient and their family. SCI is often thought of as one of the most severe types of injury, resulting in dramatic changes to all aspects of the individual's life and having a significant impact on their family and friends. Unless health care professionals have specific training or experience of SCI they are often fearful of providing care and treatment, because of the legitimate concern of causing further trauma. This chapter aims to provide an evidence-based review of the rehabilitation of SCI patients, and indicative content includes:

- Incidence and aetiology of SCI
- Function of the spinal cord and systems
- Patient assessment and management at various stages of their journey through the health care system
- Sexual issues
- Risk management of potential complications

Incidence and aetiology of SCI

In the UK, the incidence of spinal cord injury was estimated by Harrison (2000) at 500–700 people per year. However, this figure may be misleading as Cardine (1994) has suggested that the potential for spinal cord injury is always present in a patient who has sustained trauma to the vertebral column . . . any patient with injury above the clavicle or any patient unconscious after trauma.

Harrison (2000) reported that the most frequent form of SCI, within the UK, is from a rapid, unforeseen impact or deceleration. Therefore one could propose the likelihood for SCI is the same after a fall at home as it is after a road traffic accident (RTA). Helling *et al.* (1999) estimated that the majority of patients presenting with SCI (28% of the population) had experienced a low fall at home. These authors described a low fall as one that is less than 6 metres in height. Moreover, they believe this cause of injury is poorly appreciated in most regional trauma centres.

Morris & Lavery (2004) state that, 'a missed cervical injury has been associated with 10 times the rates of neurological complications'. They highlight the five techniques that may be used to exclude spinal cord injury:

- Clinical signs and symptoms
- Plain radiographs
- Computed tomography (CT)
- Magnetic resonance imaging (MRI)
- Dynamic fluoroscopy

Morris & Lavery (2004) affirmed the Advanced Trauma Life Support (ATLS) Guidelines from the American College of Surgeons, which states that:

'For patients who are comatose, have an altered level of consciousness, or are too young to describe their symptoms: all such patients should have at least a lateral and AP c-spine x-ray. Whenever possible, an open-mouth view should also be obtained. If the entire c-spine can be visualised and is found to be normal, the collar can be removed after an appropriate evaluation by either a neurosurgeon or orthopaedic surgeon . . . when in doubt leave the collar on, a cervical CT scan can be obtained somewhat later.'

Complications resulting from prolonging the duration of immobilisation and collar wearing cannot be underestimated and are explored further in this chapter. The most frequent causes of injury as illustrated by Harrison (2000) are:

- Forced hyperextension injury (e.g. falling up or down stairs)
- Forced flexion injury (e.g. head-on RTA)
- Compression injury (e.g. diving into a swimming pool/jumping from height)
- Flexion/rotation movements (during deceleration)

Many terms are used to describe a spinal cord injury, most of which are inaccurate. 'Dissection', 'transection' and 'cutting' are frequently used to describe the injury. This is not usual, unless the patient has experienced a penetrating trauma to the spinal cord. The correct term is 'spinal lesion'. A spinal lesion occurs when there is ischaemic necrosis to the area, either due to direct blunt trauma or bruising to the spinal cord. Harrison (2000) states that, 'the resulting oedema and vascular damage start a complex series of physiological and biochemical reactions within the spinal cord'. Physiological and biochemical changes set off what can be described as a chain reaction of events. As the amount of swelling increases around the spinal cord the cord is compressed, again disrupting the nerve impulse pathway.

There are two types of spinal cord injury: complete and incomplete. In a complete injury, the spinal cord is damaged across the whole of its width. This means that there is no function, either sensation or muscle control, below the level of the injury. It also means that both sides of the body are equally affected. An incomplete injury does not spread across the whole of the spinal cord: some areas away from the injury remain intact or intact enough to retain some function. Those who have an incomplete injury have some sensation and/or movement control below the level of injury. Often one side of a person's body is more affected than the other.

Function of the spinal cord and systems

The spinal cord is approximately 45 cm in length and is divided into 31 different segments, corresponding with 31 pairs of spinal nerves. The spinal cord has a central canal, surrounded by grey matter, which in turn is surrounded by white matter (Martini, 2001). The grey matter contains the cell bodies of neurons, neuroglia (glial cells) and unmyelinated axons. The greatest quantity of grey matter is located in the segments that manage the sensory and motor control of the limbs. Grey matter is organised into two groups: sensory and motor nuclei. The sensory nuclei relay the signals sent from peripheral receptors and the motor nuclei issue motor commands to peripheral effectors (Tortora & Grabowski, 2000). The white matter contains large numbers of myelinated and unmyelinated axons. It is the myelination of most of the axons that gives the white matter its colour. Each spinal segment has an association with the dorsal root ganglia, which contain the cell body. Lying laterally to the dorsal root ganglia are the spinal nerves, which are classed as mixed nerves as they contain both sensory (afferent) and motor (efferent) nerve fibres. Efferent fibres transmit outgoing messages and afferent fibres transmit incoming sensory data.

The autonomic nervous system (ANS) enables automatic control at a subconscious level of vital functions, for example blood pressure, heart rate, body temperature, appetite, gastrointestinal motility and sexual function. The organs that are served by the ANS receive two supplies of nerves: the parasympathetic nervous system, which originates from neurons in the craniosacral region of the central nervous system; and the sympathetic nervous system, which originates from the thoracolumbar region of the spinal cord. Despite the fact that the parasympathetic and sympathetic nervous systems frequently have opposite effects on an organ, their work is integrated to ensure the correct response from that organ.

The parasympathetic section of the ANS takes charge of everyday functions, such as elimination, digestion and conservation of body energy. Stimulation of this system results in an increase in peristaltic movement and a decrease in heart rate. The sympathetic nervous system is responsible for the 'fight or fight' response. If this system is stimulated the heart rate is increased and blood is shunted from the viscera to the cardiopulmonary circulation. Acetyl-choline is an important element in the chemical transmission of a message to both systems.

As specialist nurses in rehabilitation it is important that we have a firm understanding of the anatomical structures of the spinal cord, because that enables us to calculate which muscles will be affected linked to an exact area of damage to the grey matter. This will assist the multidisciplinary team in identifying the exact extent of the damage caused by the SCI, and facilitate an accurate rehabilitation programme to be developed in partnership with the patient and their family.

Patient assessment and management

Smith (2005) has stated that the key points relating to the management of a patient with an SCI in the acute stage are that:

- An SCI is a multisystem and life-changing event for the individual.
- The long-term outcome is directly affected by the quality of the care/ treatment within the first 48 hours after injury.
- Early referral to a specialist spinal centre is essential to maximise outcome and minimise complications for the patient.
- Health care professionals working in acute settings, such as the emergency department, must be adequately trained in the management of SCI, including normal and altered neurophysiology.

At the site of injury

Any patient who has sustained an injury should receive the primary assessment of airway, breathing and circulation. If the patient with a suspected SCI is unable to maintain their own airway then the responder must perform the jaw thrust, chin lift to ensure patency of the airway, and thus enable the patient to receive adequate oxygenation and perfusion. It must be stressed that any unnecessary movement of the head and neck, especially flexion and hyperextension, should be avoided.

The patient's head and neck should be examined to identify any obvious abnormality of the spinal cord. If at all possible, the entire spine should be examined for additional deformity, haematomas and localised pain; however, this is not always possible. Following a rapid examination of the patient's thorax and abdomen to assess for associated injuries, the patient's neck should be immobilised. In fact, the goal is total spinal immobilisation.

A conscious patient with a paralysis will usually be able to identify pain at the site of injury, because the loss of sensation is below this level. On examination, the patient may indicate pain through verbal and non-verbal signals and the examiner must be vigilant for these signs. It is important to consider that an associated injury within the abdomen or thorax below the level of injury may be masked by loss of sensation and paralysis.

If the patient is unconscious, then clinical findings that indicate a spinal injury are:

- Flaccid areflexia, especially with flaccid rectal sphincter
- Diaphragmatic breathing
- Ability to flex, but not extend at the elbow
- Grimaces to pain above but not below the clavicle
- Hypotension with bradycardia, especially without hypovolaemia
- Priapism, an uncommon but characteristic sign

Shock following spinal cord injury is a common feature. The examiner will have to consider all types of shock if the patient has been involved in a severe trauma. Neurogenic and spinal shock affects patients with spinal cord injuries.

Neurogenic shock occurs from impairment of the descending sympathetic pathways in the spinal cord. This results in a loss of vasomotor tone and loss of sympathetic innervation to the heart, which causes pooling of intravascular blood and results in a profound hypotension. As a result of loss of cardiac sympathetic tone, the patient may be unable to become tachycardic or even bradycardic. Thus this is not a true hypovolaemia and the examiner will need to be aware that any aggressive fluid resuscitation will only result in the patient becoming fluid-overloaded (Grundy & Swain, 2002).

Spinal shock refers to the neurogenic condition that occurs shortly after the injury. As there is little room for swelling within the limits of the vertebral canal, the oedematous spinal cord is quickly squashed against the surrounding vertebral bone. Tissue necrosis rapidly occurs as the free blood flow and oxygen within the spinal cord is disturbed. This is termed 'spinal shock' (Harrison, 2000).

Spinal shock can persist for up to six weeks following injury. It is a major factor in the patient's early rehabilitation and is often poorly appreciated in the way it affects the internal systems. Hardy & Elson (1976; cited in Harrison, 2000, p. 19) stated that:

'The management of a spinal cord injury with tetraplegia or paraplegia is difficult because within every one patient there are various, equally important, conditions to be treated. None of these must be neglected and in no field does the concept apply more forcibly of treating patients as a whole. It is for the purposes of description only that it is necessary to consider separately the various features of the clinical picture. The practical management encompasses all details, and naturally, it is only in spinal injury centres where experience in looking after so many aspects of the case at once is likely to be found.'

So what is the practitioner looking for in the assessment and diagnosis of spinal shock? Cardiovascularly, the effects of spinal shock are extreme vasodilation and flaccidity of the muscles beneath the level of the lesion. Harrison (2000) highlighted the fact that parasympathetic nervous activity remains unaffected by a spinal cord injury so cardiac output is dominated by vagal activity. Usually the patient will present with a bradycardia of around 50–60 beats per minute. The practitioner must be cautious if the patient re- quires tracheopharyngeal suctioning as overstimulating the vagal nerve during the suctioning procedure can lead to cardiac syncope and possible arrest. If the patient is in arrest, then care will need to be exercised regarding the volume of fluid used in resuscitation. This is because the patient may not have a true hypovolaemia and over-fluid resuscitation can lead to other complicated respiratory complications, such as pulmonary oedema and the systemic inflammatory response syndrome (SIRS). If cardiac compression is required, the person who is responsible for the patient's airway management will also have to prevent unnecessary movement of the spinal cord during cardiac compression, which is particularly difficult to achieve during a crisis. It should be noted that patients with spinal cord injury often have a condition known as 'poikilo- thermia'. This is due to the temperature control mechanisms becoming affected: through the inability to vasodilate or vasoconstrict, the patient essentially becomes 'cold blooded' and mimics their surrounding environmental temperature.

Transfer to the critical care unit

If the patient is conscious they will have high psychological needs: they may experience varying degrees of anxiety, stress, pain and disorientation. The practitioner will need to be aware that, although there is a vast volume of work to do in the initial phase of admission, the priority to the patient is reassurance and information. It cannot be stressed enough that the patient must be informed and consent to all procedures and investigations. If the patient is unconscious then the practitioner may still be able to communicate with the patient through touch and speech – it is well documented that hear- ing is the last sense to go.

On admission to the critical care unit, the patient will receive a more detailed examination than was conducted within the emergency department, as time will be able to be spent on a detailed neurological examination and evaluation. One of the main assessments on arrival to the unit is whether the patient's neurological status has improved or deteriorated during the transfer from the A&E department. Hughes (1997) advocated that the most useful tool in the assessment of neurological status and function is the Glasgow Coma Scale (GCS) scoring system. It is important to remember that all SCI patients may suffer spinal shock at any time and the neurological function of the patient may rapidly deteriorate, so detailed monitoring of the patient is vital to adjust care and therapy at the point of the patient's need. Assessment when the patient arrives onto the unit also allows the practitioner to establish a baseline from which all comparisons of function can be measured. The neurological assessment of a patient's coma level will comprise three main assessments:

- **Glasgow coma scale**
  - — eye opening
  - — motor response
  - — verbal response
- **Brainstem function**
  - — pupillary reactions
  - — corneal responses
  - — spontaneous eye movements
  - — oculocephalic responses
  - — oculovestibular responses
  - — respiratory pattern
- **Motor function**
  - — motor response
  - — muscle tone
  - — tendon reflexes
  - — seizures

Patients who have a lighter grade of coma will still be able to respond verbally. However, the practitioner should be aware that there has been a direct link between many of the incidents which have led to a spinal cord injury and alcohol and drugs. Therefore this factor should be looked for and identified within the emergency department or within the critical care unit, as both of these could have a profound effect on the patient's neurological condition. In addition, there is the possibility that either substance will mask the patient's true neurological function. Sequential recording of the patient's neurological state will enable a clearer picture of the patient's condition to emerge. This will facilitate early medical or surgical intervention, should the need arise.

The patient, as previously discussed, will have had their neck immobilised, usually through the application of a hard collar. The most common type used within our area of practice is a Philadelphia collar. It allows the patient's neck to be correctly sized and also has the added advantage of comprising two parts, which makes its application to the patient easier.

A patient within the critical care unit will require multiple investigations at regular intervals to adjust ongoing therapy. When the patient has become physiologically stable enough they should be transferred to a centre for spinal injuries so that optimal rehabilitation can begin.

Transfer from critical care to a spinal injuries' centre

Transfer from the acute care area to rehabilitation can be a very frightening experience for some patients. Many patients who leave the critical care environment suddenly feel very alone and isolated, as the nurse to patient ratio may be very different. Patients should be informed of their transfer well in advance to enable them to rationalise and digest the information. If transfer to the spinal injuries' centre is rushed, or not discussed and negotiated with the patient and their family fully, this can lead to agitation and anxiety. The Trust in which this author is employed is extremely fortunate to have a consultant nurse in spinal injuries, and it is this nurse who liaises with the patient and their family whilst they are in the critical care unit. The development of an early therapeutic relationship is very important to minimise anxiety about the transfer to the spinal injuries' centre. The specialist nurse uses this opportunity to reinforce the positive aspects of the step down in care and the benefits of rehabilitation and the road to independence. Family and friends can play a key role in this, but they themselves must have the support and faith in the staff to believe that this is the right thing for the patient. Transfer to a spinal injuries' centre within the UK can mean a long distance from the patient's home, as there are only thirteen specialist spinal injury units within Great Britain and Northern Ireland. The specialist nurse has a vital role to play in supporting and preparing the patient and their family for transfer to the spinal centre. Once the patient's condition has stabilised and they have been transferred to the specialist rehabilitation centre, the process of coping with a spinal cord injury becomes salient. Barry Corbet (1980; cited in Trieschmann, 1988, p. 65) encapsulated the heart of the problem as a patient, stating:

> 'One dilemma was obvious: to cope or not to cope. To cope meant to work and play and live and love as if nothing had happened. Not to cope meant to refuse responsibility for personal health and welfare, to allow physical and psychological complications to bankrupt rehabilitation. Suicide was even considered, and nobody knew for sure if that was coping or not coping. All the options seemed lousy.'

For further discussion on the levels of psychological support we can offer as specialist nurses, please refer to Chapter 4. Sexuality is often a subject that members of the health care team feel embarrassed to discuss with patients and their partners, as noted in Chapter 4. However, for the patient with an SCI it is very important that they are given permission to discuss sexuality and sexual activity in a safe and confidential environment.

Sexual issues

Many issues, which would not normally be an issue, present themselves following a spinal cord injury. Issues surrounding altered body image and others' perception of the injured person become apparent. None is more apparent in the days and weeks following injury than that of the issue of sexuality. The Spinal Injuries Association (2002) has highlighted that rediscovering one's sexuality post-injury is often another challenge the injured person will have to come to terms with, and that self-esteem and confidence will have a major role to play. The Spinal Injuries Association (SIA), (2002) advocated that a patient must reclaim his or her own body as a good first step. This is because many patients have felt that, post-injury and within the ward environment, their body is no longer their own as nursing and medical staff have access to the genital area for the purposes of hygiene and catheterisation. The SIA (2002) has recommended that maintaining an autonomous approach will enhance any relationships with a partner.

Just because someone has had an SCI it does not mean there will be any changes in their sexual preferences or attitude towards sex. Those who had a negative attitude towards sex are unlikely to change post-injury, similarly those who had a liberal sexual outlook are unlikely to change. Past experiences and beliefs will influence how patients respond to exploring their own sexual needs. The role of the specialist nurse is to reassure the patient that it may take weeks, months or years for them to feel ready to start the process of rediscovering their own sexuality. A barrier to this rediscovery is the level of anxiety the patient may have in terms of their physical ability, and how their partner will perceive them. Issues surrounding bodily functions, such as spasm during intercourse or incontinence, may cause a great deal of anxiety. The SIA (2002) have found that through thorough discussion and preparation partners are prepared and that a spinal cord injury need not interfere with sex.

Many aids, equipment and treatments are widely available to the injured to enhance their sexual enjoyment, including Eros-CTD (clitoral therapy device) for women and vacuum assistance devices and Viagra for men. The specialist nurse will be able to discuss, at length, whatever aid is used with both the injured person and their partner, should they wish. At this author's specialist Trust, patients have the opportunity to discuss all their sexual needs with the consultant nurse prior to discharge. This nurse can offer expert advice on this sensitive subject and provide a resource list.

Risk management of SCI patients

A number of medical complications and emergencies present as a real threat to the SCI patient, both within tertiary rehabilitation and the patient's home environment, and cannot be ignored. All those involved with the patient's care must be aware of the potential risks and be proactive in evidence-based risk management. Complications include: deep vein thrombosis (DVT); autonomic dysreflexia; paralytic ileus; and pressure sores. Discussion of presenting signs and symptoms and prophylactic measures is provided below.

Deep vein thrombosis

Thumbikat *et al.* (2002) emphasised that deep vein thrombosis (DVT) and pulmonary embolism (PE) in the SCI patient is not uncommon. In fact, the SIA (2002) reported that DVT occurs in 60–100% of those with a spinal cord injury; hence, all SCI patients receive DVT prophylaxis.

Alexander *et al.* (2002) discussed the fact that clot formation is more likely to occur when blood flow within the veins is reduced. Clot formation can be due to a variety of elements including obstruction and stasis, but is also due to an augmented blood viscosity, sluggish flow and damage to the endothelial wall of the vessel. Hypercoagulability is a feature of dehydration and possible underlying malignant disease. The nurse caring for SCI patients must keep a detailed account of the patient's fluid balance. A detailed past medical history is also required, either from the patient or the next of kin. Stasis lets clotting, which would usually be cleared from the circulation, continue for longer. Usually, the muscles of the legs pump together with the negative intrathoracic pressure during inspiration to promote a venous return; however, an SCI annihilates this action, thus predisposing the patient to stasis of the venous circulation. This is why SCI patients are at greater risk of DVTs than other patients. The risk also increases if the patient has had to undergo surgery, as the muscle relaxants administered during surgery abolish the muscle pump and breathing is under positive pressure when a patient is mechanically ventilated.

Thumbikat *et al.* (2002) discovered, through their own research at The Princess Royal Spinal Injuries Unit in Sheffield, that there were two peak periods of venous thromboembolism: the first at 20–30 days following injury and the second at 90–100 days post-injury. They found that the severity of associated injuries did not result in a higher incidence of DVTs, although those who had sustained cervical injuries appeared to be more prone to venous thrombosis than those with lower spinal injuries.

Identification of DVTs becomes even more difficult in the SCI patient as one of the symptoms is calf pain and tenderness, particularly on dorsiflexion. There are other signs that will indicate a DVT, for example the calf may be red and swollen or the patient may present with pyrexia. During the first few months post-injury all patients will have to wear anti-embolism stockings, as well as undergoing frequent passive lower limb movement and regular repositioning. Repositioning the patient with SCI may be difficult; however, the use of turning beds and kinetic therapy beds may be useful. The nursing staff may also measure the patient's calves for a comparison.

Pharmacological intervention will also be required, in the form of heparin, warfarin or enoxaparin, if a DVT is detected and as prophylaxis against further clots.

Autonomic dysreflexia

This is a possible life-threatening condition. Autonomic dysreflexia (AD) is an exaggerated response of the nervous system to a localised trigger, usually below the level of the spinal cord injury. Tomassoni and Campagnolo (2003) have recognised AD as a 'syndrome of massive imbalanced reflex sympathetic discharge occurring in patients with [an] SCI above the splanchnic sympathetic outflow (T5–T6)'. An AD trigger could be anything, but is often due to an overfull bladder or bowel. The irritated or painful area attempts to send messages or signals to the brain via the spinal cord; however, due to the injury, the messages are unable to reach the brain. The activated response or reflex increases the activity of the sympathetic portion of the autonomic nervous system. This reaction involves constriction of the vessels in the skin and abdomen. As constriction occurs, the pressure within the vessels rises; it is this mechanism that causes a massive, and rapid, hypertensive episode.

The most concerning feature about this phase in the condition is the potential to experience a cerebrovascular accident (CVA), seizure or even death. However, the body does mount counteroffensive measures. During AD the body attempts to compensate for the hypertension through vasomotor brainstem reflexes increasing parasympathetic stimulation to the heart via the vagus nerve, causing a compensatory bradycardia, and attempts to vasodilate the vessels. It is this response that causes the person with AD to have such severe headaches.

Some of the signs and symptoms of AD

- Hypertension
- Pounding headache
- Sweating above the level of injury
- Bradycardia < 60 beats per minute
- Blotching of the skin – mainly across the chest
- Cool, clammy skin below the level of injury
- Nausea
- Anxiety
- Restlessness

If the patient experiences any of these symptoms you must sit the patient up or raise the head of the bed **immediately**. (Sitting the patient up counteracts the rise in BP with orthostatic hypotension.) This is a life-threatening situation. Call for help as soon as possible. Look for causes of irritation, such as:

- Full, blocked, kinked catheter bag; signs of a urinary infection
- Tight clothing; sharp objects in any pockets
- Evidence of pressure sores, cuts, burns, bruises and ingrown toenails
- Overdistended bowel, through constipation/impaction
- Infection of the bowel through infection or irritation, e.g. appendicitis
- Overstimulation during sexual activity
- Menstrual cramps
- Acute abdominal conditions
- Skeletal fractures

The cause of irritation must be resolved and emergency medical treatment must be sought if the condition persists.

Bladder and bowel management

Many health care professionals do not consider bowel management to be a priority of care for the acute spinal injured patient. However, for the patient this may become a life-threatening condition, for instance as a contributing factor in autonomic dysreflexia, perforation of the intestine or an acute abdomen. Immediately post-injury there will be an episode of paralytic ileus. A paralytic ileus is something that all SCI patients experience and it is vital to remember to keep the patients nil by mouth for at least 48 hours post-injury during this phase, regardless of whether bowel sounds are heard or not. This is because a paralytic ileus may occur during the phase of spinal shock. Obviously, the nutritional status of the patient will need to be considered carefully if an ileus persists after 72 hours, and it may be necessary to commence total parenteral nutrition (TPN).

The anal reflex is one of the first reflexes to return post-injury (usually within the first 48 hours), although patients with a lesion below the level of T12 will not recover this reflex due to the involvement of the corda equina (Harrison, 2000). It is important for the patient to develop a bowel programme early on in their care. This will ensure that the patient is participating in the care and management of their own bowels: to do this, it is useful for the patient or carer to maintain a bowel diary.

Manual evacuation may be necessary. This can be achieved using glycerol (glycerin) suppositories to soften the stool, the glycerol also acts as a rectal stimulant because of its mildly irritant action (British National Formulary, 2005). It is vital to patients' long-term care that only the mildest of pharmacological preparations are used during their initial care, as there will be very little choice left 10 years later if bowel cleansing preparations are used in the early phase. This procedure is often considered to be an extended area of practice; however, most trusts have readily available courses. If you have any doubt it is advisable to contact your nearest spinal injuries unit for specialist advice.

Tissue viability

Care of the SCI patient's skin is a priority to prevent pressure sore formation. In the acute phase, whilst the patient is in A&E, it is important to gain cervical clearance as soon as possible to enable the patient to be removed from the spinal board. Often, patients spend an unnecessary amount of time on hard spinal boards for a number of reasons, such as waiting for the consultant spinal surgeon to clear the neck, delays in the X-ray or CT department, or often through the department's inexperience.

Pressure sore formation starts the moment the patient is injured and is caused by the lack of sensation and movement. Pre-injury, people make instinctive movements to ensure free movement, to ensure a free circulation of blood and to prevent pressure damage to the skin and surrounding muscles and tissue. This ability is lost following an SCI (Spinal Injuries Association, 2002).

Alexander *et al.* (2002) concurred with Banks' (1992) definition of a pressure sore as 'an area of localised damage to the skin and may involve underlying structures. Tissue damage can be restricted to superficial epidermal loss or extend to involve muscle and bone'.

The National Pressure Ulcer Advisory Panel (NPUAP) (1992) has devised a four-stage classification of pressure sores, as advocated by Reid & Morrison (1994) in their work to attempt some level of standardisation of degrees of damage to the tissues:

Stage 1: non-blanchable erythema of intact skin.
Stage 2: partial thickness skin loss involving the epidermis and possibly also the dermis.
Stage 3: full thickness skin loss involving damage or necrosis of subcutaneous tissue, which may extend down to, but not through, the underlying fascia.
Stage 4: full thickness skin loss with extensive destruction, tissue necrosis or damage to muscle, bone or supporting structures.

What can be done to avoid pressure sore formation? Quite simply the answer is repositioning the patient frequently. How often depends on the individual needs of the patient. Harrison (2000) has advocated that two-hourly turning for pressure relief remains the optimal practice for the relief of pressure areas. He concurs with a plethora of other authors in that the recommended two-turning techniques are: log rolling for patients with thoracolumbar injuries, although this method of turning may be contraindicated in some cases of spinal abnormality or ridigity; and the pelvic twist for patients with cervical injuries.

An electric or kinetic profile bed may be used when it is impossible to turn the patient manually, either because of poor staffing or the patient being unable to tolerate manual turning due to multiple injuries. However, caution must be used as the patients will only be able to be turned 20–30 degrees. This is because it is impossible to ensure that a patient who is paralysed will remain in their lateral spinal position against gravity if turned beyond this angle. During the acute phase of their care, all patients are nursed in bed naked. This is to prevent them from lying on any creased clothing, buttons or zips, which may all contribute to the development of a pressure sore. A tabard may be placed over the patient to protect their dignity. It is vital to remember that the patient will feel very exposed and care will be required to maintain the patient's dignity at all times.

Conclusions

This chapter has discussed the multifaceted nature of the role of the specialist nurse in the rehabilitation of people with SCI. In-depth skills and knowledge are required in the risk management of potential complications, systematic assessment and psychological support for the patient and their family. Early transfer to a specialist spinal centre is very important once the patient's condition has been stabilised.

References

Alexander P., Fawcett N. and Runciman P.J. (2002) *Nursing Practice; Hospital at Home*, 2nd edn. London, Churchill Livingstone.

Banks V. (1992) Pressure sores: a community problem. *Journal of Wound Care*, **1** (2), 42–44.

British National Formulary (2005) *Antiplatelet Drugs*. London, British Medical Association, p. 119.

Cardine N.L. (1994) *Emergency Care on the Streets*. Boston, Little, Brown & Co.

Corbet B. [Cited in Trieschmann R. (1988) *Spinal Cord Injuries: Psychological, Social and Vocational Rehabilitation*, 2nd edn. New York, Demos Publications, p. 65.]

Grundy D. and Swain A. (2002) *ABC of Spinal Cord Injury*, 4th edn. London, BMJ Publishing Group.

Hardy A. and Elson R. (1976) *Practical Management of Spinal Injuries: A Manual for Nurses*, 2nd edn. Edinburgh, Churchill Livingstone.

Harrison P. (2000) *Managing Spinal Injury – Critical Care – the Initial Management of People with Actual or Suspected Spinal Injury in High Dependency and Intensive Care Units*. London, Spinal Injuries Association.

Helling T.S., Watkins M., Evans L.L., Nelson P.W., Shook J.W. and Van Way C.W. (1999) Low falls: an underappreciated mechanism of injury. *Journal of Trauma, Injury, Infection and Critical Care*, **46**, 453–456.

Hughes R. (1997) *Neurological Emergencies*, 2nd edn. London, BMJ Publishing Group.

Martini F. (2001) *Fundamentals of Anatomy and Physiology*, 5th edn. Upper Saddle River, N.J., Prentice Hall.

Morris C.G. and Lavery G.G. (2004) The unconscious trauma patient: cervical injury or not? *Journal of the Intensive Care Society*, **5** (1), 22–25.

National Pressure Ulcer Advisory Panel (1992) *Statement on Pressure Ulcer Prevention*. www.npuap.org

Reid J. and Morrison M. (1994) Towards consensus: classification of pressure sores. *Journal of Wound Care*, **3** (3), 157–160.

Smith M. (2005) Care of patients with acute spinal cord injuries. [Cited in Kneale J. and Davis P. (2005). *Orthopaedic and Trauma Nursing*, 2nd edn. Edinburgh, Churchill Livingstone, p. 362.]

Spinal Injuries Association (2002) *Moving Forward 3: The Guide to Living with Spinal Cord Injury*. London, SIA.

Thumbikat P., Poonnoose P.M., Balasubrahmaniam P., Ravichandran G. and McClelland M.R. (2002) A comparison of heparin/warfarin and enoxaparin thromboprophylaxis in spinal cord injury: the Sheffield experience. *Spinal Cord*, **40**, 416–420.

Tomassoni P. and Campagnolo D. (2003) Autonomic dysreflexia: one more way EMS can positively affect patient survival. *Journal of Emergency Medical Services*, **28** (12), 46–51.

Tortora G. and Grabowski S. (2000) *Principles of Anatomy and Physiology*, 9th edn. New York, Wiley.

Chapter 12
The Way Forward

Rebecca Jester

This concluding chapter aims to draw together the salient points of the preceding chapters, and to discuss some of the key issues for succession planning in terms of preparing the next generation of nurses to specialise within rehabilitation. Also, there is a need for us to support ourselves and each other in our roles to further advance nursing practice in rehabilitation through robust systems of dissemination of evidence-based practice. The indicative content of the chapter includes:

- Implications for advancing nursing practice
- Education and training for advancing practice
- Mentorship
- Clinical supervision
- Action-learning sets
- Evidence-based nursing

Implications for advancing nursing practice

The need for nurses to advance their practice in rehabilitation has never been more pressing than at the present time. Demographically, the increase in the number and proportion of older people, and/or those with chronic long-term conditions, has necessitated a major redirection of service delivery within the UK. Specifically, new ways of working are evident in the increasing shift toward primary care-led services, with more home-based rehabilitation and the implementation of case management and self-management for those with complex comorbid conditions. Also, legislation has affirmed that society should provide an enabling environment for those with disability and that they have the right to equitable rights and treatment. Recognition has been affirmed for informal carers, and we are now required by legislation to provide assessment, support and services for them as well as those they care for. National service frameworks for older people and those with long-term conditions require health care providers to meet national standards, including improved partnership working with patients and their families, increased choice and rehabilitation delivered by those with specialist skills and knowledge. In response to these new developments, an ever-increasing number of advancing practice roles have been developed, for example nurse consultants and advanced nurse practitioners. It is essential that those advancing their roles are prepared and supported to work at a higher level if the roles are to be effective. This requires innovative and flexible approaches to learning and teaching, and systematic approaches to ongoing support for practitioners.

Education and training for advancing practice

Frequently, the terms 'education' and 'training' are used interchangeably within health care settings. However, they are not the same. Rather than providing an analysis of educational theory to differentiate between the two, I will share with you a quote from a former tutor of mine. He stated that: 'education and training were not the same and whilst he was happy for his fourteen-year-old daughter to undergo sex education he was not happy for her to undertake sex training'. When preparing to advance our practice we often need a combination of education and training. Furthermore, some basic principles should underpin this preparation, as outlined in Table 12.1.

As recommended by the Department of Health (1999), those aiming to advance their practice need to be educated to post-graduate level. However, there has been little guidance from the professional bodies regarding what should be included in an educational programme to prepare nurses to advance

Table 12.1 Principles of preparation for advancing practice roles.

- Leadership and role negotiation are imperative to the success of advancing practice roles
- Preparation should comprise both generic and individualised learning components
- Interprofessional learning should be maximised
- Learning outcomes should be linked into the key skills framework (KSF) wherever possible
- The individual learner will need the full support of their employing organisation both during and on completion of the period of study
- Learning should be linked into skills-based commissioning for the rehabilitation service they are employed within
- Preparation will require both education and training and a combination of both classroom and clinically based learning opportunities
- Learners will need to be supported by both an academic and a clinical facilitator
- Following completion of a programme of study the practitioner will need to undertake activities such as clinical supervision or action learning sets to facilitate continuing professional development
- Learning should be flexible and include various approaches such as distance learning, work-based learning and be based upon the principles of adult learning

their roles; except that to be eligible for a specialist practitioner qualification the programme of study should comprise both theory and practice in equal distribution. Through my own experience of developing and evaluating post-graduate curricula in advancing practice, I have found there are a number of key subjects that should be included, which are:

- The sciences underpinning practice – applied anatomy/physiology/pathophysiology, psychology and sociology
- Advanced holistic health assessment
- Leadership
- Role development and negotiation, including management of change
- Clinical decision-making
- Legal and ethical aspects of advancing practice
- The application of research to improve practice
- Pharmacology and prescribing
- Service evaluation and outcome measurement

This list is not meant to be exhaustive, but rather an outline of core curriculum content. Opportunities for accreditation of both prior accredited learning and experiential learning should be maximised to avoid unnecessary repetition for learners and to value previous learning. The curriculum should endorse the principles of adult learning. Knowles (1984) identified six assumptions made about adult learning:

- Relevance – adults need to know why they need to know something
- Self-concept – students seen as being capable of self-direction
- Experience – adults have a wealth of experience upon which to draw for their learning
- Readiness to learn – adults are motivated to learn what is relevant to them at that moment
- Orientation to learning – motivation is enhanced when new learning is perceived as helping them to deal with problems they meet within their real-life roles
- Motivation – internal motivation in terms of increased job satisfaction and self-esteem

Methods of delivering the curriculum must endorse these assumptions about how adults learn. To do this, a variety of learning and teaching methods is required, for example: work-based learning, negotiated learning using learning contracts (please refer to Chapter 6 for further detail); experiential learning through observation and supervised practice; and the use of problem-based curricula. These are all examples of formal learning methods; however, a significant part of learning related to advancing our practice constitutes informal learning in the workplace.

Informal learning

Many health care professionals equate learning with formal education and training and assume that working and learning are two separate activities that never overlap. However, Eraut (2004) suggested that: 'most workplace learning occurs on the job rather than off the job' (p. 249). Informal learning is largely invisible and often not recognised as legitimate learning by the individual or their organisation. Eraut (2004) has distinguished between levels of informal learning as follows:

- Implicit learning – the acquisition of knowledge independent of conscious attempts to learn.
- Reactive learning – brief reflection in action, where we make a mental note of facts, ideas, impressions and the recognition of possible future learning opportunities.
- Deliberative learning – there is a definite learning goal and time is set aside for the acquisition of new knowledge.

When aiming to advance our practice it is highly desirable to utilise all three components of Eraut's typology of informal learning. Specifically, deliberative learning activities should be maximised and include methods such as mentorship, clinical supervision and action learning sets.

Mentorship

Mentorship has been defined as 'help by one person to another in making significant transitions in knowledge, work or thinking' (Megginson & Clutterbuck, 1997; p. 13). This suggests that mentorship should be non-hierarchical and not aligned to line management. Effective mentorship for those learning toward advancing practice roles is absolutely essential. A number of key issues to address related to mentorship include:

- Who should mentor advancing practice students?
- How should mentors be prepared for their role?
- What qualities are we looking for in an effective mentor?

Finding a suitable mentor is crucial to maximise success in preparing for advancing practice roles. A mentor should have both the aptitude and willingness to take on the mentorship role, and have sufficient time and resources to support the learner. Mentors may come from a variety of professional backgrounds, but should have the relevant skills and knowledge in both the specialist area (rehabilitation) and in supporting and challenging the learner. The balance between providing the right amount of support and challenge to the student is crucial, too much support and not enough challenge will result

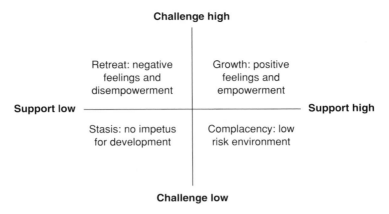

Fig. 12.1 Relationship between challenge and support. Adapted from Daloz (1999).

in understimulation of the student, and probably underachievement; too much challenge and not enough support can lead to the student feeling threatened and distressed (Daloz, 1999). Fig. 12.1 provides a useful illustration of the relationship between support and challenge in mentorship.

There are a number of potential advantages and disadvantages to seeking mentors from professions other than nursing; one of the advantages being to resolve the present scarcity of suitably qualified and experienced advanced practitioners working within rehabilitation nursing. Politically, it may be advantageous to choose a mentor who has power and influence within the organisation, because, as discussed in Chapter 2, the development of advancing roles may well meet with some resistance. Based upon my own students' experiences they have received good quality mentorship from practitioners from a variety of professional backgrounds in rehabilitation, including: consultant medics; superintendent physiotherapists; clinical psychologists; and nurses already established in advanced practice roles. In addition to identifying a main mentor, it is advantageous to have a number of associate mentors to give support for distinct aspects of the student's learning goals. Quality mentorship requires commitment and time. In addition, teaching and learning activity in the clinical setting needs to be skilfully negotiated to contribute to the planned learning. The type of activities that facilitate learning will include observation of the mentor or associate mentor when they are treating rehabilitation patients, and then moving along a continuum of confidence until the student can practise under supervision from the mentor/s. Time for personal reflection on observation and supervised practice is a key element for learning, as is time spent with the mentor engaged in critical analysis of clinical events using skilled questioning as a vehicle for learning and development.

One of the practical difficulties for nurses studying to advance their practice is being able to disengage from their previous role within the organisation. For example, when participating in clinical learning events with their mentor the student may be called upon for advice and support on other matters. Clinical learning time must be protected: students often find it useful to change to a student uniform and an identity badge that states they are a post-graduate student. These visual reminders to team members, in addition to briefing colleagues on the requirements of your clinical learning, should assist in minimising interruptions. Students often express anxiety about 'embarrassing themselves' in front of their clinical mentors with whom they may have had a long-standing professional relationship.

The academic facilitator has an important role in preparing mentors for their role to ensure the student is provided with a safe learning environment. Workshops provide an interactive medium to prepare and support mentors for their role, as they will be able to meet and network with other mentors. Mentors need to be supported in their role and feel empowered to discuss any difficulties they are encountering with the academic team. Mentors often worry about 'failing' students, especially if the student is a colleague they like and respect. Issues such as this should be included in the mentor preparation workshops, and there should be regular review meetings between the mentor, their student and the academic facilitator to discuss the student's progress.

Clinical supervision

In addition to the initial preparation for an advancing practice role, practitioners are continually required to update their skills and knowledge to ensure their patients receive evidence-based quality care. One approach adopted within heath care to facilitate ongoing personal and professional development is clinical supervision. It is important to differentiate between managerial supervision, which is generally hierarchical and associated with the appraisal and monitoring of employee performance, and clinical supervision, which has been defined as: 'A supportive relationship that provides a focus for shared learning, developing and restoring self, and identifying learning needs' (Fowler & Chevannes, 1998; p. 380).

The supportive and developmental focus of clinical supervision is affirmed by Proctor's (1986) work detailing three functions of clinical supervision, which are formative, normative and restorative tasks. The shared tasks of supervision as identified by Proctor (1986) are summarised in Table 12.2.

Some of you may have participated successfully in clinical supervision for a number of years, but there are still a significant number of individual practitioners and health care organisations that have not effectively established clinical supervision. In part, this may be due to the inherent difficulty of evaluating the impact of clinical supervision on clinical outcomes in the context of a health service struggling with burgeoning costs and finite budgets. However, there is a considerable body of evidence to support the positive impact of clinical supervision for organisations, including: improved staff well being and performance; reduced stress; reduced sickness; improved staff retention;

Table 12.2   The shared tasks of supervision (Proctor, 1986).

Formative: (development)	Developing skills and enhancing understanding, building on practitioner's abilities, enabling personal and professional development.
Normative: (assessment)	Shared responsibilities for monitoring standards and the ethical practice of the practitioner, through self-assessment and valuing contributions.
Restorative: (refreshment and creativity)	Relating to the affective or emotional domain, allowing for the sharing of feelings and discharging and recharging of emotions and energies.

and a workforce that is attuned to lifelong learning (Butterworth *et al.*, 1997). Wilson & Palmer (1999), from their evaluative studies, also reported a number of positive benefits and outcomes of clinical supervision for individual practitioners, which included:

- Encourages sharing of ideas between practitioners and enhances patient care
- Facilitates better team-working
- Encourages reflection on practice
- Allows exploration of alternative approaches to care
- Promotes better communication
- Provides a more focused service to patients
- Increases professional support
- Helps increase practitioner's confidence
- Helps combat stress

There are various models of clinical supervision, including group, one to one and live supervision. Choosing the right model depends on a number of factors unique to the individual practitioner as there are potential advantages and disadvantages inherent to each model, as summarised in Table 12.3.

Planning and implementing clinical supervision requires support from all levels of the participating organisation, from the senior executive group to the individual practitioners. Individuals must be adequately prepared to engage in clinical supervision as supervisors and/or supervisees. Those engaging in clinical supervision must have prerequisite skills in: self-awareness, reflection, active listening, critical analysis and problem-solving to be effective in both the roles of supervisor and supervisee. As discussed in the context of mentorship, one of the important issues for a supervisor is achieving the right balance between challenge and support, which is referred to as the 'warm bath' and 'cold shower' aspects of clinical supervision. Whichever type of clinical supervision is decided upon, the ground rules should be formalised in a contract between the participants. These should include issues such as confidentiality and when confidentiality may be breached to maintain patient safety or if serious

Table 12.3 Summary of potential advantages and disadvantages of types of clinical supervision.

Type of clinical supervision	Potential advantages	Potential disadvantages
One to one	• Confidentiality may be more assured. • Easier to arrange meetings between two individuals	• Some individuals may be uncomfortable with the intensity of one-to-one challenge.
Group	• Benefit from collective expertise of group. • Some individuals may feel safer within a group.	• Meetings can be difficult to coordinate. • Group dynamics can adversely affect the supervisory process.
Live	• Particularly useful when there may be issues of poor self-awareness for the supervisee.	• Some individuals may find the process intrusive to themselves and their patients.

misconduct is reported. Specifically, those working in rehabilitation may find multidisciplinary group supervision beneficial to enhance an individual's awareness of the profession-specific and shared issues they are encountering as a team. Clearly, clinical supervision is not the only method of promoting lifelong learning in health care, and action-learning sets have gained momentum in the UK, specifically for those developing advancing roles in practice.

Action-learning sets

Action learning, a process of learning and reflection, is facilitated by the support of a 'set' of colleagues, working on real issues, with the intention of getting things done (McGill & Brockbank, 2004). Action learning is defined as:

'An approach to individual and organisational development. Working in small groups, people tackle important issues or problems and learn from their attempts to change things.' (Revans, 1998; p. 32)

This approach is ideally suited to advance practice within rehabilitation, because it recognises the importance of collective problem-solving and that the process of working together is as valuable as the outcomes achieved. An isolated individual is unlikely to make a significant impact on advancing practice if not supported by their colleagues and the organisation *per se*. Therefore action learning can provide a vehicle for development not only for the individual advanced practitioner, but for the whole rehabilitation team. The participants in the 'set' learn with and from each other, and take forward an important issue with the support of the other members of the set. Action learning builds on the relationship between reflection and action. As with clinical supervision, prerequisite skills of self-awareness, reflection, active listening, critical analysis and problem-solving are required by all set members for action learning to be effective.

The action-learning process should again be a balance between support and challenge, while recognising the unique contexts and experience individuals bring to the set. Developing and sustaining an action-learning set takes careful preparation, commitment and support. Set members should be recruited on a voluntary basis; it is useful to ask an experienced facilitator to run a 'taster session' for potential set members so they can gain a better insight into what will be involved. The ethos of action learning is based upon giving greater emphasis to the acquisition of questioning insight, rather than an overreliance on accumulated knowledge (Revans, 1998).

Advancing practice requires not only initial educational preparation, but ongoing personal and professional development. Clinical supervision and/or action learning are tools that can support this. As an individual and as a rehabilitation team it is important to explore these methods and decide what will meet your individual and collective needs most suitably. Advancement of practice and ongoing development are essential to the delivery of contemporary evidence-based rehabilitation practice. Commissioners of rehabilitation services will require evidence that your service is cost-effective, evidence-based and meets the recommendations of national and local guidelines. As an advanced nurse practitioner it is essential that you are able to effectively evaluate various types of evidence to underpin and advance patient care.

Evidence-based nursing

Background

Despite the fact that evidence-based nursing did not gain widespread adoption until the 1990s, nurses have been using research to underpin their practice since the nineteenth century:

> 'In dwelling upon the vital importance of sound observation, it must never be lost sight of what observation is for. It is not for the sake of piling up miscellaneous information or curious facts, but for the sake of saving life and increasing health and comfort.' (Florence Nightingale, 1859)

During the Crimean war, Florence Nightingale collected data on morbidity and mortality rates of wounded soldiers and analysed the data to ascertain if there was a relationship between delay to operating time and post-surgical survival.

The genesis of evidence-based nursing practice is, in part, a response to the

Table 12.4   Types of evidence (adapted from Le May, 1999).

- Evidence from research – carrying out a search of published and unpublished literature and using systematic reviews. Including guidelines and protocols developed using empirical evidence
- Evidence based on experiences – reflecting on practice and using non-research publications such as case studies to facilitate discussion on best practice
- Evidence based on theory that is not research based – formal education, symposia and conference presentations
- Evidence gathered from clients and/or their carers about issues of satisfaction/dissatisfaction/complaint and audit data about untoward incidents

need to provide cost-effective, high-quality care (DH, 1996). Ritualistic practice is no longer acceptable. Whilst not all nurses are academically prepared to undertake research, all nurses must have an awareness and appreciation of research and how to implement appropriate findings into their everyday practice.

Defining evidence-based practice and what constitutes evidence

Evidence-based nursing is described by Sackett *et al.* (1996) as nursing decisions based on:

- Best available evidence
- Value of clinical experience
- Patient preference

This suggests that nurses can use evidence from a number of sources to underpin their practice. A summary of the types and sources of evidence can be found in Table 12.4.

In recent years, a number of organisations have developed resources to assist practitioners in developing evidence-based practice via systematic reviews, databases and best practice guidelines. Examples include: The Cochrane Library, incorporating the Cochrane Database of Systematic Reviews, the Cochrane Controlled Trials Register and the Cochrane Review Methodology Database; the Midwifery Information and Resource Service (MIDIRS); NHS Centre for Reviews and Dissemination; and literature searching facilities such as Medline, Psyclit and the Cumulative Index of Nursing and Allied Health Literature (CINAHL).

It must not be assumed that all research, guidelines and publications in professional journals are valid and reliable. Nurses must be able to critically review evidence to assess its validity before basing their practice upon it. A summary of the questions to ask about research papers to ascertain their validity can be found in Table 12.5. DiCenso *et al.* (1998; p. 38) suggested that:

Table 12.5 General questions to ask about research papers (adapted from DePoy & Gitlin, 1994).

- Was the study clear?
- Was the research question or hypothesis clearly stated?
- Was the rationale for the study identified?
- Did the research design and methods fit the purpose?
- Was the literature review relevant and systematic?
- Were the threats to reliability and validity acknowledged and controlled?
- Were the methods of analysis clear and appropriate?
- Do the findings address the research question or hypothesis?
- Are the implications for practice acknowledged?
- Do the conclusions fit with the data presented?
- Are ethical considerations discussed?
- Who undertook the research?
- Who funded the work?
- Do you have enough information to repeat the study?

'in practising evidence based nursing, a nurse has to decide whether the evidence is relevant for the particular patient. The incorporation of clinical expertise should be balanced with the risks and benefits of alternative treatment for each patient and should take into account the patient's unique clinical circumstances, including co-morbid conditions and preferences.'

An example of the application of the above quotation is the use of full-length, anti-embolic stockings in preventing deep vein thrombosis following lower limb surgery, e.g. total hip replacement. However, in taking into account the patient's individual needs we may discover that the patient either has a comorbid state that prohibits the use of anti-embolic stockings or finds them so uncomfortable that the patient rolls them down, increasing the risk of vascular complications. This example demonstrates the necessity for nurses to view evidence-based practice in the context of individual holistic nursing care.

Potential barriers to implementing research-based practice and types of support available

Nurses may encounter barriers to implementing evidence-based practice, including:

- Negative staff attitudes – lack of motivation, resistance to change, fear and ritualised practice.
- Organisation issues – time, resources, pressure of work and too much change.
- Educational issues – unable to access research, lack of knowledge and skill in research appraisal, language of research makes it inaccessible.
- Cooperation issues – medical colleagues may block implementation, other professions believing nursing research is substandard.

It is important to remember you are not alone in the struggle to implement evidence-based practice and that seeking support and guidance is essential. To overcome potential barriers and to maximise success in the implementation of evidence-based practice there are many opportunities for support, including:

- Organisational support – trust-based research and development units, enhanced links with higher education, specific appointments (trust-based research experts and lecturer practitioners) and availability of literature searching databases.
- Support structures – research forums within the trust and specialist interest groups, journal clubs and ethics committees for nursing research.
- Educational support – study days, conferences, workshops and distance learning packages to develop skills in utilising research.
- Interprofessional support – opportunities for multiprofessional research, multidisciplinary team approach to guideline and protocol development.

Conclusions

This concluding chapter has attempted both to demonstrate approaches to initial preparation for advancing nursing practice roles and methods of personal and professional continuing development. The importance of evidence-based practice has been affirmed in the context of the need to consistently demonstrate the effectiveness of our services to commissioners, patients and their families.

A summary of the different evidence sources that may be used to underpin practice has been provided, and the need to balance the use of evidence and individual patient need emphasised. Use of research necessitates the ability to differentiate between valid and poor evidence sources, and a brief guide to critiquing research has been presented. Potential barriers to implementing evidence-based practice have been identified and a variety of support systems and resources highlighted to help nurses succeed in using evidence to improve patient care.

References

Butterworth T., Carson J., White E., Jeacock J., Clements A. and Bishop V. (1997) *It is Good to Talk: An Evaluation Study in England and Scotland. Clinical Supervision and Mentorship Series*. University of Manchester, School of Nursing, Midwifery and Health Visiting.

Daloz L.A. (1999) *Mentor. Guiding the Journey of Adult Learners*. San Francisco, Jossey-Bass Publishers.

Department of Health (1996) *Promoting Clinical Effectiveness: A Framework for Action in and Through the NHS*. Leeds, NHSE.

Department of Health (1999) *Making a Difference: Strengthening the Nursing, Midwifery and Health Visiting Contribution*. London, DH.

DePoy E. and Gitlin L. (1994) *Introduction to Research. Multiple Strategies for Health and Human Services*. St Louis, Mosby.

DiCenso A., Cullum N. and Ciliska D. (1998) Implementing evidence-based nursing: some misconceptions. *Evidence-based Nursing*, **1** (2), 38–40.

Eraut M. (2004) Informal learning in the workplace. *Studies in Continuing Education*, **26** (2), 247–273.

Fowler J. and Chevannes M. (1998) Evaluating the efficacy of reflective practice within the context of clinical supervision. *Journal of Advanced Nursing*, **27**, 379–382.

Knowles M. (1984) *The Adult Learner: A Neglected Species*. Houston, Texas, Gulf Publishing.

Le May A. (1999) Evidence-based practice. *Nursing Times Monographs, No 1*. London, Nursing Times Books.

McGill I. and Brockbank A. (2004) *The Action Learning Handbook: Powerful Techniques for Education, Professional Development and Training*. London, Taylor and Francis Routledge.

Megginson D. and Clutterbuck D. (1997) *Mentoring in Action*. London, Kogan Page.

Nightingale F. (1859) *Notes on Nursing*. Philadelphia, J.B. Lippincott.

Proctor B. (1986) A cooperative exercise in accountability. In: *Enabling and Ensuring* (M. Marken and M. Payne, eds). London, Council for Education and Training in Youth and Community Work.

Revans R. (1998) *ABC of Action Learning*. London, Lemos and Crane.

Sackett D., Rosenberg W. and Muir Gray J. (1996) Evidence-based medicine: what it is and what it isn't. *British Medical Journal*, **312** (7023), 71–72.

Wilson A. and Palmer A. (1999) *Making Clinical Supervision Work: The Evaluation Report*. Middlesex, Harrow and Hillingdon Healthcare NHS Trust.

Further reading

Morton-Cooper A. and Palmer A. (2000) *Mentoring, Preceptorship and Clinical Supervision*, 2nd edn. Oxford, Blackwell Science.

Index